Recent Research in Psychology

Mary L. Pritchard

Psychological Aspects of Rheumatoid Arthritis

Springer-Verlag
New York Berlin Heidelberg
London Paris Tokyo Hong Kong

Mary L. Pritchard
Department of Psychology
Washington Singer Laboratories
University of Exeter
Exeter EX4 4QG
United Kingdom

With 4 Illustrations.

Library of Congress Cataloging-in-Publication Data
Pritchard, Mary L.
Psychological aspects of rheumatoid arthritis / Mary L. Pritchard.
p. cm.—(Recent research in psychology)
Includes bibliographical references.
1. Rheumatoid arthritis—Psychological aspects. I. Title.
II. Series.
[DNLM: 1. Arthritis, Rheumatoid—psychology. WE 346 P961p]
RC933.P697 1990
616.7'227'0019—dc20 89-21615

Printed on acid-free paper.

Camera-ready copy provided by the author.
Printed and bound by Edwards Brothers, Inc., Ann Arbor, Michigan.
Printed in the United States of America.

9 8 7 6 5 4 3 2 1

ISBN 0-387-97116-5 Springer-Verlag New York Berlin Heidelberg
ISBN 3-540-97116-5 Springer-Verlag Berlin Heidelberg New York

For Mom, Dad and Andy

PREFACE

The main research described in this book is concerned with assessing the interrelationship of psychological adjustment, compliance with medical advice and use of unorthodox treatments in a sample of rheumatoid arthritic out-patients. Basically this research is comprised of four components: two pilot studies; the development and postal administration of an illness knowledge assessment questionnaire; and a 'follow-up' correlational study.

Pilot study 1, which involved interviews with 18 patients, was a 'question seeking' study - the aim being to develop research questions of relevance to the subject sample. The findings of this study suggested that poor illness knowledge and consequent misconceptions was contributing to psychological distress and affecting health behaviour among patients.

In pilot study 2 a sample of 17 patients were questioned in detail - but using open-ended questions - about their understanding of their condition and treatment. The results of this study supported the impression gained in pilot study 1, that patients were typically ill-informed about their illness and tended, in the absence of correct information, to overestimate the risks associated with rheumatoid arthritis and underestimate the value of treatments.

This latter study also identified a number of specific misconceptions patients held about rheumatoid arthritis and these were incorporated into a multiple-choice illness knowledge assessment questionnaire, which was then sent to a sample of 170 rheumatoid arthritics living in Exeter and outlying areas - 128 usable replies were obtained. Following item and factor analysis of the data obtained from this and a second sample of 114 patients (from Torbay) a 27 item multiple-choice questionnaire was 'arrived at'.

Seventy-five of the Exeter patients (randomly selected) who had returned questionnaires were followed-up with interviews, for what comprised the main study. In these interviews patients were questioned about their use, experience, and evaluation of conventional medical treatments and unorthodox treatments; and their emotional reactions to rheumatoid arthritis. Additionally patients completed a pain locus of control scale

(BPCQ); the General Health Questionnaire; the McGill Pain Questionnaire and a series of visual analogue pain scales; and a disability assessment index. Basic demographic and illness history data was also collected.

Factor analysis of this data revealed a core of five/six main factors. These were concerned with: physical and psychological distress; non-compliance with conventional medical treatment; use of 'home' or personally supervised unorthodox treatments; use of faith related unorthodox treatments or intrapsychic coping stategies; and there was also a factor which most probably reflects the quality of the doctor-patient relationship and on which loaded, among other things, ratings of conventional medical treatment, illness knowledge, socio-economic status, and use of unorthodox practitioners.

The best correlates of psychological distress were pain, the 'chance' scale of the BPCQ, and ratings of the helpfulness of conventional medical treatment. Correlates of compliance included helpfulness ratings of conventional medical treatment, socio-ecomonic status and depression.

Use of 'home' unorthodox treatments appeared to reflect a need for self-help and involvement. Use was greatest amongst female patients; was positively associated with anxiety, minding taking conventional medical drugs, the practice of exercise, and duration of illness; and was negatively associated with depression, pain variability, and a 'powerful other' locus of pain control orientation.

Female patients were also more likely to use faith related unorthodox treatments (e.g. prayer, faith healer). Other variables associated with the use of faith include: illness knowledge, age, ratings of conventional medical treatment, and the experience of benefits as result of having rheumatoid arthritis. Unorthodox practitioner use was also negatively associated with ratings of conventional medical treatment, but in contrast to the use of faith, was negatively associated with illness knowledge. Users of unorthodox practitioners (chiropractors and acupuncturists) also tended to be of lower socio-economic status than non-users, and have higher 'chance' and 'internal' locus of pain control scores.

ACKNOWLEDGEMENTS

I should like to thank all the patients who participated in this research, and Dr Richard Jacoby, their consultant, for their cooperation and affability. Thanks also to members of the Social Work, Physiotherapy, and Occupational Therapy departments at the Princess Elizabeth Orthopaedic Hospital for their help.

I am also grateful to many people in the department of Psychology at Exeter University, for their advice and guidance, but in particular to Mr Keith Nichols and Professors J. Richard Eiser and Paul Kline.

Finally, I wish to thank Andy, my Mother and Father, and friends, especially Marie, for their forbearance, encouragement and support.

This research was funded by the Medical Research Council.

CONTENTS

CHAPTER 1

INTRODUCTION

RHEUMATOID ARTHRITIS

Rheumatoid arthritis (RA) is a condition affecting around 2% of the population and accounting for almost 10% of visits to G.P.s (Logan and Cushion, 1958). Two-thirds of those affected are women and although RA can affect people of any age it most commonly strikes in the early-middle years and post-menopausally (in women).

RA is a systemic inflammatory disease primarily affecting the synovial joints. Involvement of other body organs and systems (such as the heart, blood vessels, alimentary tract, lymph nodes, bone marrow, skin, muscles and peripheral nerves) although quite common, does not invariably occur and often, when it does, is clinically asymptomatic.

The major symptoms of RA are those of inflammation, namely: localized pain, stiffness swelling and heat; pyrexia; and general malaise. Deformity can also occur but is typically not a presenting symptom. Certain deformities such as the 'ulna drift' - where the fingers 'lean' towards the ulna bone - are particularly characteristic of RA.

The 'seat' of pathology in the rheumatoid process appears to be the synovial membrane, which becomes hypertrophied and inflamed and produces an abnormal tissue, pannus, which grows over the articular cartilage, eroding it and eventually the underlying bone (see Figure 1.1). RA is often described as being an auto-immune disease as much of the joint damage is thought to be caused by the action of enzymes released from immune cells (e.g polymorphonuclear leucocytes) involved in the inflammatory process. Mechanical degradation of bone tissue probably also occurs later in the disease process as a result of the articular surfaces, devoid of their layer of cartilage, rubbing. This damage is compounded by osteomalacial changes which are accelerated in RA. The joints also suffer mechanical damage as a result of 'soft' joint structures (e.g. tendons, joint capsule) being permanently stretched and, hence slackened by the swelling inside the joint

Figure 1.1

Comparison of a normal and rheumatoid arthritic joint.

(Diagrams taken from the Handbook for Patients (1985) and reproduced by kind permission of the Arthritis and Rheumatism Council of Great Britain)

(a) a normal synovial joint

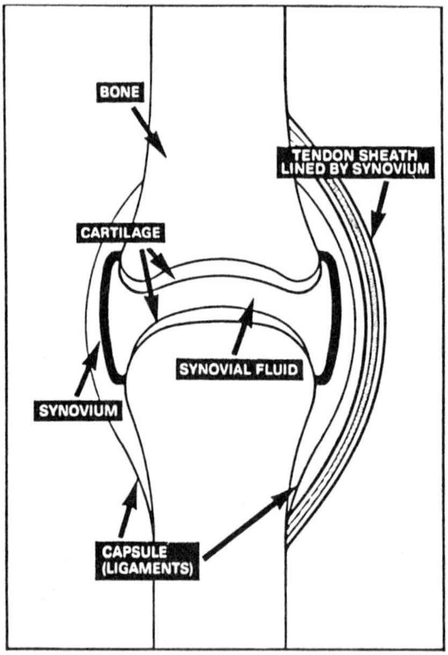

(b) the synovial inflammation of RA

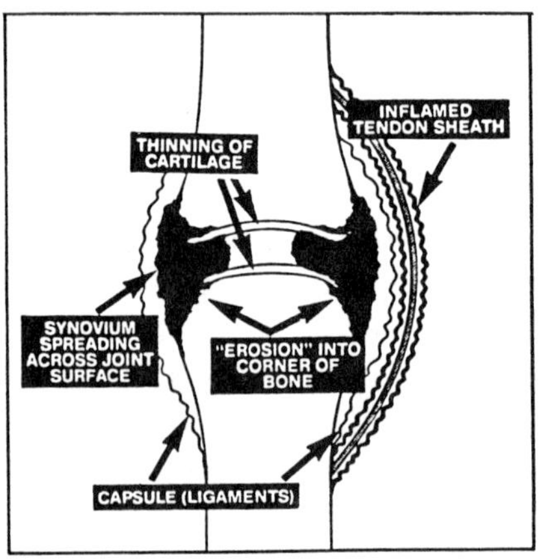

Prognosis and Disease Course

Which joints and body systems become affected and how badly varies very much from patient to patient. For some people their RA represents nothing more than a mild twinge now and again. In other cases severe disability and even mortality (Reah, 1963) can result. The statistics available regarding disability prognosis are not very consistent. This probably reflects the use of vague and different criteria. Thus Huskisson and Hart, (1978) suggest that less than 10% of sufferers become 'completely disabled' and 50% ultimately suffer 'little or no disability', while the Arthritis and Rheumatism Council (ARC, 1985) suggests that around 5% of sufferers 'develop severe disease with extensive disability' while 30% 'recover completely within a few years' and 65% 'continue having joint pain, swelling and flare-ups'. These differences may also reflect recent improvements in treatment or differences in patient inclusion criteria. It has been suggested that around 50% of patients attending a hospital out-patient department for their RA might expect to develop 'severe functional incapacity ' within 10-15 years of first being seen (Ragan and Farrington, 1962).

Typically the disease is marked by periods of exacerbation ('flare-ups') followed by periods of remission. In some cases, however, as already mentioned, the disease can remit completely and in others it can be unremitting or 'malignant'. Overlaying the interpersonal and intrapersonal variability the tendency is for the disease to become less aggressive with time.

Treatment

There is no cure for RA, although the contemporary utilization of more aggressive treatments early on in the course of the illness means that the above estimates of disability probably represent overestimates. Four main types of medical treatment are available for RA: drugs, surgery, physiotherapy and occupational therapy.

A variety of surgical procedures have been used in RA. At one time removal of the synovial membrane was undertaken as an aggressive 'preventive' treatment in early RA. Lately, however, this procedure has fallen from favour and surgery in RA is now primarily reparative, palliative or undertaken to restore function - e.g. joint replacements, arthrodesis, tendon repairs.

Four main categories of drug are used in the treatment of RA: analgesics, steroids, non-steroidal anti-inflammatory (NSAI) drugs and disease modifiers. The mainstays are NSAIs and disease modifiers. Ideally NSAI drugs (e.g. aspirin, ibuprofen) should obviate the need for analgesics as reduction of inflammation will relieve pain. They are also to be preferred over analgesics. As mentioned above, much deformity and loss of function is caused by the stretching and consequent slackening of 'soft' joint structures such as the joint capsule and tendons. Use of inflamed and swollen joints makes this damage much more likely to occur, hence there is a need to avoid reduction in pain (which will encourage joint use) without concomitant reduction in inflammation. Steroids, although they may produce a very dramatic reduction in patient symptoms do not appear to affect the underlying disease process or progression, and may aggravate joint destruction via osteomalacial changes. They are also undesirable in view of other side-effects. Finally, disease modifiers are those drugs which appear to suppress the disease process. They include: anti-malarial drugs such as the chloroquines; cancer drugs such as azathioprine; penicillamine; and gold. Although the mode of action of these drugs is generally poorly understood it is known that they do not have any direct analgesic or anti-inflammatory action.

The role of physiotherapy and occupational therapy in the treatment of RA is to minimize 'mechanical' joint damage and maximize functional capacity and personal independence. Specifically, the occupational therapist (OT) and physiotherapist may: devise exercises to restore joint function and prevent function loss; advise on home exercise programmes and the use and protection of joints; provide patients with personalized splints; and devise ways in which patients can overcome daily living problems.

The physiotherapist is likely to instruct RA patients in two main types of exercise: 'range of motion exercises' and 'strengthening exercises'. The former as their name suggests involve moving the joints through their full range of motion. The idea is to prevent the loss of movement and, hence, function of the joint. Strengthening exercises are aimed at building and toning the muscles supporting the joints and involved in movement. They again are important in maintaining function and may also protect the joint from mechanical damage by bolstering and maintaining joint support. Special care must be taken to avoid damaging the joint and consequently exercise must be gradually built-up. Although medical opinion differs as regards the acceptability of the experience of any additional pain or discomfort following exercise, all would concur that it should not last for longer than an hour after exercise is stopped. Particular care must be taken with the very inflamed and 'active' joint. At one time such joints were put in casts to immobilize them, now it is thought they should ideally be put through their range of motion twice daily to preserve mobility. It is thought rest at such times serves to prevent some joint damage and reduces the duration of acute 'activity'.

Advice about the way to use joints and the availability of special devices or aids is important both in terms of protecting the joints from further damage and in terms of maintaining the patient's independence. For example, right-handed patients may be advised, when cooking, to stir in an anti-clockwise direction and left-handed patients to stir clockwise. Similarly, patients may be advised to not rest their hands on their hips or rest their forehead against their hands. All this advice is directed at avoiding the 'ulna drift' deformity. A general piece of advice is to use the largest joint possible, for example, the elbow to close tin lids.

Finally, joint splints for a variety of joints, including the neck, knees, hands and wrists may be prescribed. Most common is the wrist splint of which there are two types: day splints and night splints. The function of both is to protect the joint from 'mechanical' damage. Day splints may also serve, by supporting the joint, to aid function.

Cause

The cause of RA is not really understood. A variety of hypotheses have been tendered over the years but at present the most popular is that RA is the result of a genetic immune vulnerability in association with a viral/bacterial 'trigger'.

PSYCHOLOGICAL ISSUES IN RHEUMATOID ARTHRITIS

The psychological research literature on RA is somewhat limited, being predominantly comprised of attempts to assess the validity of the 'psychosomatic hypothesis' - the notion that psychological stress or personality variables can cause physical illness. The research questions addressed in this book rather than being initially derived from this literature were derived from an exploratory 'question seeking' study (pilot study 1). The results of this study are outlined in greater detail in Chapter 5, at this juncture suffice it to say that the findings of pilot study 1 highlighted a number of issues worthy of further study, namely:

(1) psychological distress in rheumatoid arthritics (RAs);

(2) compliance with medical advice;

(3) use of unorthodox treatments; and

(4) illness knowledge.

Uniting the first three topics is the issue of patients' illness knowledge. The impression gained in the pilot study was that a lack of knowledge was contributing to psychological distress, non-compliance and possibly unorthodox treatment use.

PLAN OF THE BOOK

Chapters 2 to 4 are reviews of the relevant research literature. Specifically, Chapters 2, 3, and 4 are concerned with the determinants of psychological distress, compliance/non-compliance and use of unorthodox treatments respectively. In each case research with RAs is supplemented by a consideration of other relevant research. Many questions and hypotheses addressed in the following research were developed from a consideration of this research literature and are outlined in these review Chapters. Chapter 5 describes pilot study 1, mentioned above. Two studies concerned with establishing what RA patients understand about their illness are described in Chapter 6. Chapter 7 is the methodology Chapter for the main study, the results of which are presented and discussed in Chapters 8 through 10. Finally, the last Chapter concludes with a discussion of some of the most interesting findings and their practical implications.

CHAPTER 2

PSYCHOLOGICAL DISTRESS IN RHEUMATOID ARTHRITIS

INCIDENCE AND NATURE OF DISTRESS

There is a fairly substantial and consistent body of research indicating that levels of psychological distress or disturbance are elevated in people suffering from RA (see Anderson et al, 1985; and Achterberg-Lawlis, 1982, for reviews).

Gardiner (1980), for example, reports significant psychiatric disturbance - using the 30 item General Health Questionnaire (GHQ; Goldberg, 1967) - in 53.5% of his sample of British rheumatoid arthritics (RAs). This morbidity, he notes, is significantly higher than population norms. Goldberg and Huxley (1980), summarizing a variety of studies, note psychiatric morbidity prevalence rates of between 9% and 24% in the general population. In a British sample, using the GHQ, Goldberg et al (1974) found a prevalence rate of 18.4%.

Depression

As to the qualitative nature of the reaction, there is much evidence to indicate that it is depressive in nature. Studies using a variety of psychometric instruments, including the Minnesota Multiphasic Personality Inventory (MMPI; Hathaway and McKinley, 1967 - Polley et al, 1970; Liang et al, 1984;, Bourestom and Howard, 1965; Spergel et al, 1978), the Beck Depression Inventory (BDI; Beck, 1978 - e.g. Rimon, 1969) and the Zung Depression Scale (SDS; Zung, 1965 - Gardiner, 1980) have consistently revealed elevated depression levels in RA samples.

In one of the earliest objective studies Rimon (1969) reports a 28% incidence of depression among 100 RA out-patients using the BDI. Studies of the General population have found prevalence rates for depression of between 5.7 and 18.3% (Goldberg, 1980) and in studies using self rating depression scales, prevalence rates of between 16 and 18% have been reported (Weissman and Myers, 1978).

In a more recent study, Liang et al (1984) found 'abnormally' high scores on the depression scale of the MMPI in 41.2% of their sample of 160 RA out-patients. The results of other studies support this higher incidence. For example, using the same scoring of the BDI as Rimon, Zaphiropoulos and Burry (1974) report evidence of depression in 46% of their sample.

Anderson et al (1985) note that depression scores have tended to be between one and two standard deviations above the mean, which they suggest indicates mild reactive depression. There is some evidence, however, that depression may be greater in RAs than in other chronically ill populations (e.g. Polley et al, 1970; Zaphiropoulos and Burry, 1974), although, other researchers have found comparable levels of depression in RA and non-RA chronically ill controls (Liang et al, 1984; Spergel et al, 1978).

Anxiety

Far fewer studies have assessed anxiety, as compared to depression, levels in RAs. Subjective clinical reports suggest elevated anxiety (see Anderson et al, 1985) as do the majority of studies that have assessed anxiety related personality traits such as: neuroticism (EPI; Eysenck and Eysenck, 1964 - Gardiner, 1980), hypochondrias, hysteria (MMPI; Hathaway and Mckinley, 1967 - Liang et al, 1984) emotionality, apprehension, worry and tension (16PF; Cattell, 1965 - Moldofsky and Rothman, 1971; and Robinson et al, 1971). Crown et al (1975), however, found no differences between female RAs and healthy controls using the Middlesex Health Questionnaire (MHQ; Crown and Crisp, 1966) which has six scales (free floating anxiety (FFA), phobic anxiety, obsessionality, somatic anxiety, depression and hysterical traits). Although, male RAs had significantly higher scores on the FFA scale.

Psychosis

Quite a few researchers have noted a low incidence of schizophrenia in RA sufferers (see Taylor, 1978; and Rimon, 1969, for reviews). One suggestion is that schizophrenia and RA represent alternative physiological reactions to psychological stress (see Taylor, 1978, for details of this and other explanations of the low coincident rate).

EXPLAINING PSYCHOLOGICAL DISTRESS IN RHEUMATOID ARTHRITIS - RESPONSE OR ANTECEDENT?

There is a substantial body of evidence supporting the notion that life stress contributes to psychiatric illness (see Cochrane, 1980). Physical illness undoubtedly represents a considerable life stress and particularly a chronic illness such as RA which potentially can, and frequently does, have a major and generally negative affect on many aspects of an individuals life, including: familial and marital relationships (e.g. Liang et al, 1984; Yelin et al, 1979; and Cobb et al, 1959); sexual functioning (Richards, 1980); work (Earle et al, 1979); and social activities (Cobb et al, 1965; and Kasl and Cobb, 1969). The suggestion that psychological stress or distress is implicated in the aetiology of physical illness, although supported by a growing body of evidence, is more contentious.

A Premorbid Arthritic Personality?

The possibility that psychological factors could be implicated in the aetiology of physical illness has excited considerable interest. For many years research effort was concentrated on attempts to find disorder specific personalities or psychological conflicts. Quite a considerable amount of research effort was spent looking for the rhematoid arthritic personality or conflict (for reviews see: Weiner, 1977; Solomon, 1981; Udelman and Udelman, 1981; Achterberg-Lawlis, 1982; and Anderson et al, 1985).

The 'RA personality' has, for example, been characterised as: obsessive or perfectionist (Cobb et al, 1959, 1965; Moos and Solomon, 1964, 1965; Muller et al, 1961; Robinson, 1957); restricted in emotional expression (Blom and Nicholls, 1954; Halliday, 1942; Ludwig, 1952; McLaughlin et al, 1953); sporty (Booth, 1937; Cleveland and Fisher, 1960; Cleveland et al, 1965; Cormier et al, 1957; Halliday, 1942; Meyerowitz et al, 1968); dependent (Alexander, 1950; Halliday, 1942; Sochet et al, 1969); aggressive (Alexander, 1950; Halliday, 1942; Ludwig, 1954); subservient, insecure and sensitive (Moos and Solomon, 1965); unconfident (Mueller et al, 1961); and hard-working and self-sacrificing (King and Cobb, 1958).

While there is clearly some consistency among researchers there is also considerable inconsistency and the quality of the majority of the research does not assist one in making sense of this literature. The major methodological problems are outlined and discussed by Anderson et al (1985), who state them as follows:

(1) vast differences across studies in theoretical orientations and assessment procedures;

(2) inattention to Ss' general medical information and demographic characteristics;

(3) heterogeneity within the RA population;

(4) excessive attention to negative personality characteristics;

(5) lack of appropriate control groups; and

(6) retrospective study design.

More recently the idea of a RA personality, and indeed of disease specific personalities in general, has been severely challenged. The conclusion most widely accepted today is that there is no specific personality profile implicated in the aetiology of RA. Evidence is available which suggests that there is a 'chronic illness personality', however, to which RAs conform (Spergel et al, 1978); but this is thought to be largely a response to illness rather than a cause. Crown and Crown (1973), for example, found very few differences in personality profiles between early RAs and controls.

<u>Preceding Life stress/distress</u>

As the idea of disorder specific premorbid personalities lost favour interest in premorbid life 'stress' or events gained momentum.

Early interview studies have shown an association of preceding life events and RA onset in 45% (Halliday, 1942), 62% (Cobb et al, 1939) and 100% (Sochet et al, 1969) of their samples. Unfortunately, as well as being retrospective, these studies also lacked a control group. Studies using control groups have variously supported (e.g. Baker, 1982) and disconfirmed (e.g. Lewis-Faning, 1950; Hart, 1979) the hypothesis. Possibly some of the inconsistency in results may result from difficulties in assessing life events (see Zimmerman, 1983). Particularly interesting because of its comparison of different methods of assessing life events, and because it used two control groups, is the study by Hart (1979). In this study RAs, depressives and healthy controls were required to indicate, from a checklist of 60, which life events they had experienced, and to rate the amount of control they felt they had over those events, their desirability and predictability. While Hart reports no differences between RAs and controls, both reported significantly fewer unanticipated and undesirable events in the five years preceding illness onset than the group of depressives.

There is some evidence to suggest that there may be important psychological differences among RAs regarding the role of psychological stress in the aetiology of their illness. Within his sample of 100 RAs, Rimon (1969) distinguished two major subgroups. In one, the so-called 'major conflict group' (MCG), life stress preceding disease onset had been accompanied by a 'distinct psychiatric or psychophysiological reaction'. In the other, the 'no-conflict group' (NCG), there had either been no preceding life events or conflicts or where there had, these had not been associated with psychological distress. These subgroups also differed in terms of their disease onset and progression; and family history - Ss in the MCG were less likely to have a relative with RA and more likely to have experienced a sudden disease onset and fast progression. Additionally, in this group exacerbations in disease activity, following a remission of one year or more, were associated with 'psychodynamic conflict', whereas in the NCG they were not.

Not surprisingly there have been no prospective studies looking at the role of 'stress' in the aetiology of RA. Gardiner (1980), however, did use a prospective design in examining the value of psychological factors as predictors of prognosis in RA. He reports that not one of the psychological variables (and they included the GHQ, EPI and SDS amongst others) was found to predict disease activity. Possibly, however, the long duration between psychological assessment and clinical follow-up (12 months) explains this negative result. There is evidence that psychological treatments (see Anderson et al, 1985) and psychotropic drugs (Rimon, 1974) can have beneficial effects on the disease. Unfortunately, the validity of these findings is questionable due to the reliance on self-reported measures of disease parameters and the lack of control groups for attention.

Routes Via Which Psychological Distress Could Affect Disease Onset and Progression

(a) Physiological Response Specificity

Just as some researchers have been interested in psychological specificity - finding a specific personality or specific conflict for different illnesses - the idea of physiological specificity has also been popular. Thus it has been suggested that hypertensives respond to stress with elevated blood pressure, migraine sufferers with hypervasoconstriction of the cranial arteries, and ulcer patients with hyperexcretion of hydrochloric acid (Roessler and Engel, 1974; Engel,

1972). Of RA it has been hypothesized that stress is converted into muscle tension which damages the joints and evidence to support this hypothesis is available (e.g. Christie, 1975; Sternbach, 1966; Moos and Engel, 1962; Walker and Sandman, 1977; Fisher and Cleveland, 1960; Taylor et al, 1982). Moos and Engel (1962), for example, found elevated electromyographic activity (EMG) levels near painful joints in RAs, relative to non-painful joints and matched joint sites in hypertensives. This higher baseline EMG activity has been replicated by Walker and Sandman (1977) who compared RAs, 'normals' and duodenal ulcer patients. Additionally, these latter researchers found that RAs showed a relatively higher increase in EMG response when presented with stressors (autopsy slides, anagram and arithmetic problems) than either of the other groups. Interestingly, this response was restricted to EMG; heart rate and electrogastric responses did not distinguish RAs from controls, although, they did distinguish ulcer sufferers, who showed greater responsivity in these systems.

Sternbach (1966) has in fact proposed a three component model to account for the emergence of physical illness as a response to stress. The evidence relating to two aspects of this model - response specificity and exposure to activating or stressful situations - has already been discussed. Evidence to support the occurrence of the third component - homeostatic inadequacy - is provided by studies which have found a relative delay in return to baseline levels of activity in the supposedly affected physiological system. Evidence of delayed recovery in EMG response in RA has been reported (e.g. Anderson et al, 1982).

Although an attractive idea, the evidence regarding physiological response specificity in RA is problematical for a number of reasons. First, in both the Andersen et al study discussed above and another study (Taylor et al, 1982) RAs have been found to exhibit greater responsivity than controls in other response modalities (e.g. electrodermal activity). Secondly, the possibility that the observed EMG effects represent a response to the disease itself cannot be ruled out. Thirdly, and relatedly, the mechanism via which increased muscular tension might instigate, either initially or subsequently, the rheumatoid process in joints is not outlined, nor is it easy to imagine. Medical and epidemiological evidence indicates that RA is not a 'wear and tear' arthritis, i.e. it is not associated with the use of joints, although the joints of paralysed limbs tend not to be affected. Finally, the specificity theory cannot explain the systemic effects of RA.

(b) The Effects of Stress on the Immune System

An alternative way in which it has been proposed 'stress' effects vulnerability to disease is via its affects on the immune system. As immune function is implicated in the pathogenic process and, additionally, a virus is believed to trigger disease onset, this route seems particularly appropriate in the case of RA.

Evidence that psychological and social stress can affect immunological function is available (e.g. Bartrop et al, 1977; Kiecolt-Glaser et al, 1984) but direct evidence that stress induced immunological changes actually increase vulnerablity to disease in humans is not (excellent reviews of this area are provided by Ader, 1981; and Udelman and Udelman, 1983).

Anderson et al (1985) report that only one study has linked psychological stress, immuno-function and arthritic symptoms in humans (Hendrie et al, 1971). These researchers assessed preceding life stress and immuno-function in a group of patients who had been suffering from polyarthritis for less than six months (Anderson et al suggests the inclusion criteria for Ss means that the majority were early RA sufferers) and in healthy controls and depressives. Although, as in the Hart (1979) study discussed above, only the depressives had experienced above average levels of premorbid stress, it was found that in arthritis patients with elevated immunoglobulin levels, life event scores were elevated.

Animal studies are also suggestive. Amkraut et al (1971), for example, found that severity of arthritis in rats, developed after inoculation with a pathogen, was increased by prior overcrowding.

The effects of stress on the immune system are believed to be mediated via the central nervous system, autonomic nervous system (ANS) and endocrine system. Traditionally, the immune system was thought to be self-regulatory but all the organs of the immune system (e.g. thymus, bone marrow, lymphatics) have since been found to be provided with ANS innervation and the lymphocytes and phagocytes have both been found to have receptors for neurotransmitters, hormones and other substances released directly and indirectly by neural tissue (Spector and Korneva, 1981). The precise effects of stress on the immune system is far from determined, however. The immune system is inordinately complex and researchers have typically looked at just one or two immune functions. There is evidence that the same stressor while increasing vulnerability to some infections can decrease vulnerability to others (see Plaut and Friedman, 1981). Similarly, Palmblad (1981) has proposed that immuno-suppression occurs only for the duration of the stressor and that for a period thereafter enhanced resistance occurs.

(c) Health Behaviour

Another way in which stress might affect disease progression is via its affect on health behaviour. The evidence available, although indirect, suggests that psychological stress is unlikely to reduce the chances of seeking medical help, rather the contrary (e.g. Shepherd et al, 1966). However, it may be that psychological distress reduces compliance with medical advice. If for no other reason this might be anticipated because of the affects of distress on cognitive functioning - the distressed patient is probably less likely to understand and remember advice (Nichols, 1984) and, hence, is more likely to be unintentionally non-compliant. On the other hand, in so much as psychological distress, especially anxiety, represents a motivating or driving force (Miller, 1948), compliance might be expected to be increased in physically ill patients who are concommitantly psychologically disturbed.

Evidence regarding compliance rates with psychotropic medication do not support the idea that the psychologically disturbed are less compliant (see Ley, 1979a). However, DeVon and Powers (1984) found that non-compliance in hypertensives was negatively associated with adjustment. With regard to RA, Carpenter and Davis (1976) report that compliers (with an exercise regimen) were slightly, but not significantly, more likely than non-compliers to accept their arthritis. Unfortunately, the validity and sensitivity of the measure of acceptance in this latter study is somewhat questionable - a social worker simply classified patients as 'accepting, non-accepting or neutral in their reaction'. There do not appear to be any other studies looking at the relationship of adjustment and compliance in RA.

PREDICTORS OF PSYCHOLOGICAL DISTRESS IN RHEUMATOID ARTHRITIS

DEMOGRAPHIC AND DISEASE RELATED FACTORS

Several studies have reported an association, or lack of one, between measures of psychological distress and demographic variables and disease parameters in RAs.

Sex

One study reports greater psychological disturbance in female RAs (Kasl and Cobb, 1969) and two suggest that gender is not associated with adjustment - depression (Zaphiropoulos and Burry, 1974) or 'psychosocial adjustment' (Earle et al, 1979). However, the reliability and validity of the measures of adjustment in the latter study - five likert type attitudinal indices of 'psychosocial adjustment', namely: family appreciation, self-esteem, isolation/loneliness, work satisfaction, and meaninglessness - are for the most part unknown. One study has suggested that male and female RAs show peak disturbance at different times during the course of their illness (Zaphiropoulos and Burry, 1974).

Age

In many ways the implications of a chronic disease are greater for the young and consequently one might expect age to be positively associated with adjustment in the chronically ill. This hypothesis has been supported in a heterogeneous sample of chronically ill patients (Westbrook and Viney, 1982) but two studies of RAs failed to find a significant association between age and depression (Rimon, 1969; Zaphiropoulos and Burry, 1974) and in the former study at least, the tendency was for depressed patients to be older.

Socio-Economic Status (SES)

Earle et al (1979) report that SES was positively associated with all five of their measures of adjustment (see above) in RAs - individuals in the higher SES groups showing better adjustment in each case. Rimon (1969), however, failed to find an association between SES and depression in RAs.

Generally speaking, social class has been found to be fairly consistently related to the development of both psychiatric illness (Brown and Harris, 1978; Dowrenwend and Dowrenwend, 1974; Rutter et al, 1975; Rutter and Quinton, 1976) and physical illness (DHSS, 1980; Townsend and Davidson,

1982; Syme and Berkman, 1976; Weiner, 1977); ill populations being comprised disproportionately of the lower socio-economic classes. Various explanations for this finding have been advanced. One suggestion - the social drift hypothesis - is that this reflects the fact that the weak (whether physically or psychologically) are less able to hold high status positions because of their illness (e.g. Goldberg and Morrison, 1963). The alternative position points to ways in which social class might act as a vulnerability/protection factor . Money, education and status can all be seen to provide ways of coping with stress and additionally, a lack of money and position in themselves can represent considerable stressors. In a particularly noteworthy study of depression, Brown and Harris (1978) found that differences in the incidence of 'provoking agents' (i.e. major life events and difficulties) and 'vulnerability factors' (i.e. low level of intimacy with spouse, loss of mother and three or more children under 14 years) explained, at least statistically, the observed difference in the incidence of depression among lower and middle class women.

Social Support

Many researchers have reported a significant interaction between life events and social support in predicting both psychological and physical illness (see Thoits, 1982, for a review). Main effects of social support have also been reported (e.g. Berkman and Syme, 1979; Brown et al, 1977; Henderson et al, 1978). With specific regard to the question of adjustment to physical illness, primary network support has been shown to be associated with enhanced adjustment among post-burn (Davidson et al, 1981), disabled (Ben-sira, 1981, 1983; Smith and Midanik, 1980) and stroke patients (Evans and Northwood, 1983). There do not appear to have been any notable studies looking at the role of social support in either the aetiology of illness or in adjustment to illness in RA, although two studies have looked for an association between marital status and adjustment in RA populations. Rimon (1969) reports that marital status was not related to depression scores in his sample of patients, while Liang et al (1984) found that married patients tended to have higher MMPI hypochondrias scores.

Explanations of the function of social support tend to converge (see for example, Cobb, 1976, House, 1981; Weiss, 1974). Weiss (1974), for example, has proposed the following 'provisions of social relationships': '(1) attachment, provided by close affectional relationships, which gives a sense of security and place; (2) social integration ..; (3) the opportunity for nurturing others .. which gives incentives for continuing in the face of adversity; (4) reassurance of personal worth, which promotes self-esteem; (5) a sense of reliable alliance; and (6) obtaining help and guidance from informal advisors when difficulties have to be resolved' (Henderson et al, 1980, p 725).

Disease Severity

One might predict that the more disabling and painful a disease the greater the distress, although several studies of chronically ill children have found maladjustment to be inversely associated with disability or disease severity (McFie and Robertson, 1973; Rodda, 1970; Sussman, 1966; Williams, 1970; McAnarney et al, 1974; Bruhn et al, 1971). The evidence relating disease severity and adjustment in RA is inconclusive.

Mindam et al (1981) reports that disease activity - measured in terms of: pain intensity, duration of morning stiffness, general feeling of being unwell, articular index, and grip strength - was positively associated with the incidence of 'psychiatric symptoms', as did Earle et al (1979). Zaphiropoulos and Burry (1974), however, failed to find an association between disease severity - assessed from a consideration of erythrocyte sedimentation rate; presence or absence of rheumatoid factor, nodules and erosions; and disability - and depression.

Possibly this latter negative result reflects the inclusion of disability in the assessment of severity. Functional capacity or disability has typically been reported as being uncorrelated with adjustment in RAs (e.g. Zaphiropoulos and Burry, 1974; Crown and Crown, 1975; Rimon, 1969; Kaplan and Kozin, 1981), although it has been found to be negatively associated with adjustment in other disabling diseases (e.g. multiple sclerosis - Matson and Brooks, 1979) and fear of disability is frequently reported by RAs (e.g. Rogers et al, 1982; Ehrlich, 1982). In all the above studies, however, functional capacity was assessed rather crudely, on a four point scale (Steinbrocker et al, 1949; American Rheumatism Association, 1959). Mindam et al (1980) , using a slightly more sensitive index of functional capacity, reports that the most disturbed patients in their sample of RAs, as well as having the most active disease, also showed the greatest decrease in performance of several daily activities. The recent availability of several sensitive, well validated and reliable self-report scales of functional capacity (Meenan et al, 1980; Fries et al, 1980; Berger et al, 1981) should make clarification of the relationship between disability and distress easier in future research.

The seeming inconsistency of the relationship between adjustment and disease severity may also reflect the differential assessment of adjustment - different emotional responses may have different determinants.

Intrapersonal Disease Variability

Great intrapersonal variability is a characteristic or RA and one which, because of its likely influence on perceptions of control, is likely to affect psychological distress. To date, however, the relationship of this variable with adjustment in RA does not appear to have been investigated.

Duration of Illness

Again, the evidence relating duration of illness and adjustment in RA is inconsistent. Crown and Crown (1975) report that psychological disturbance (assessed by the MHQ) is positively related to duration of illness, while Zaphiropoulos and Burry (1974) failed to find an association between illness duration and depression. These latter researchers, however, note that there was a tendency for depression, where it did occur, to do so early in the course of the disease in males and later on in females - the statistical significance of this finding is not reported, nor for that matter is any explanation offered. Inconsistent with both these studies, Matson and Brooks (1979) report that, in multiple sclerosis, adjustment (measured in terms of self-esteem) and illness duration are positively correlated. These latter researchers also note that nearly all adjustment took place within the first 10 years.

Again it is possible that the lack of consistency between studies reflects the use of different measures of adjustment. Alternatively it may reflect a lack of attention to absolute duration of illness in favour of relative duration.

Stages of Adjustment

The idea that in the process of adjusting to adverse events or life crises people progress through various stages has been very popular. Stages of adjustment have been identified for a variety of crises including: separation (Bowlby, 1960, 1973); bereavement or loss (Bowlby, 1961; Engel, 1962, 1964; Natterson and Knudson, 1960; Parkes, 1972); rape (Sutherland

and Scherl, 1970); physical disability (Gunther, 1969; Guttmann, 1976; Hohmann, 1975; Siller, 1969); criminal victimization (Symonds, 1975); spinal cord injury (Bray, 1978; Cohn, 1961; Weller and Miller, 1977); loss of a limb (Parkes, 1972); blindness (Fitzgerald, 1970); cancer (Gullo et al, 1974); chronic haemodialysis (Beard, 1969; Reichsman and Levy, 1972); open-heart surgery (Dlin et al, 1968); miscarriage (Zahourck and Jensen, 1973); multiple sclerosis (Matson and Brooks, 1979); and terminal illness (Nighswonger, 1971; Kubler-Ross, 1969). General models have also been proposed (Klinger, 1975, 1977; Shontz, 1965, 1975; Wortman and Brehm, 1975).

The typical sequence of stages described is: denial or shock, followed by 'anger' or 'invigoration', then depression and finally, recovery, 'adjustment' or 'acceptance'. In terms of a specific example, perhaps most relevant to RA is the model proposed by Matson and Brooks (1979) for multiple sclerosis, which, like RA, is a chronic disease marked by considerable intrapersonal variability and disability. These researchers suggest four stages of adjustment: denial, resistance (characterized by a search for treatment), affirmation (characterized by grieving for loss), and integration. However, Rogers et al (1982) have suggested that the 'progression of responses to acute life-threatening situations (shock, anger, denial, resignation, and acceptance) is usually altered in RA, mirroring the course of the disease' (p 344). For example, they suggest that, depending on the presenting symptoms and diagnostic history, some patients may be relieved when given a diagnosis of RA. Additionally, they state that feelings of 'resignation and acceptance' will tend to predominate during periods of stable disease activity, whereas, 'anger, sadness and anxiety' may recur during flare-ups. Similarly, others have suggested that individuals may experience more than one stage simultaneously; progress backwards and forwards; and skip stages (e.g Matson and Brooks, 1979; Klinger, 1975, 1977; Kubler-Ross, 1969). The extent to which a stage model can survive these modifications is clearly at issue.

Unfortunately, there is little objective evidence regarding the occurrence of stages of adjustment and certainly there is none regarding stages of adjustment to RA. The vast majority of relevant studies are subjective, descriptive or anecdotal in nature. Silver and Wortman (1980), who have reviewed this topic, report only one systematic attempt to validate some aspect of the stage model (Lawson, 1976) and this was restricted to a consideration of depression in spinal injury patients.

COPING

Lazarus' Conceptualization of Coping

By far the most comprehensive and useful conceptualization of coping is that developed, over a number of years, by Lazarus and colleagues (e.g. Coyne and Lazarus, 1980; Lazarus , 1966, 1974, 1981; Lazarus et al, 1974; Folkman et al, 1979) who have defined coping as, '.. efforts, both action-oriented and intrapsychic to manage (i.e. master, tolerate, reduce, minimize) environmental and internal demands and conflicts among them, which tax or exceed a person's resources' (Folkman et al, 1979, p 283).

Lazarus refers to his model as an 'interactive' or 'process' theory of coping. A key aspect in this process is 'appraisal'. Lazarus distinguishes two types of appraisal: primary and secondary. The extent to which a person experiences psychological stress is a function of both primary and secondary appraisal. Primary appraisal is where the individual assesses whether they are in fact in trouble or not. There are three basic categories of primary appraisal. A situation or event can be evaluated as being: benign and positive, irrelevant for well-being, stressful. Stressful appraisals take three forms: harm-loss, which refers to damage that has already occurred; threat, which refers to harm-loss that has not yet occurred but is anticipated; and challenge, which refers to an anticipated opportunity for mastery or gain. Secondary appraisal is where the person assesses what can be done about the situation, i.e., the adequacy, suitability and availability of coping strategies. The theory is 'interactive' because secondary appraisal will affect primary appraisal - if a problem is easily avoided or ameliorated, then it does not represent much of a problem.

According to this theory no one coping stategy (e.g. denial) is intrinsically better than any other. The best coping strategy will depend on the individual/environment interaction and is likely to change as the situation unwinds. Good coping is assessed in terms of the 'goodness of the fit among task demands, coping resources and personal agendas', where the latter refers to 'personal values, sources of meaning and well entrenched styles of thinking and acting' (Folkman et al, 1979, p 288). Put another way, in any stressful situation multiple values are at stake and by implication good coping involves the optimization or harmonization of these. Three values common to most stressful situations are: (1) the instrumental aims or goals of the situation; (2) the control of emotional reactions - maintenance of emotional homeostasis; and (3) the maintenance of feelings of self-worth and morale. Lazarus does not consider the possibility of there being a trait of good coping but in terms of the theory a good coper would be a person who manages to optimize the achievement of these three values across different situations.

Two main functions of coping strategies are distinguished. Problem-focused, or instrumental coping, as its name suggests is directed at the management of the person-environment relationship - the source of stress - while emotional-focused coping is directed at the regulation of the emotional response to the stressor. Research indicates that in most coping episodes both types of coping are used (Folkman and Lazarus, 1980). Realistic, problem-focused coping has often been assumed to be superior to emotional-focused coping (e.g. Freyberger, 1980). However, according to Lazarus, evaluation can only be made on the basis of the effect of the strategy on long (e.g. physical illness) and short-term (e.g. upset) outcomes; neither type of coping is inherently superior.

Theoretically, each type of coping can facilitate or impede the other. There is evidence to suggest that problem solving behaviour is inefficient under conditions of high emotional distress (see Hamilton, 1975, for a review of this evidence), but solving the problem is likely to be the most effective way of reducing distress. Some forms of emotional-focused coping can preclude the use of problem-solving strategies, for example, when denial of symptoms leads to a delay in seeking medical help. Ignoring emotional-focused coping, however, especially when problem-focused coping is not very effective, may similarly be damaging; the relationship of the Type A behaviour pattern - which is characterized by a problem-solving/striving approach to life - and coronary artery disease (e.g. Rosenman et al, 1975) is testimony to the need for balance.

The four main modes of coping strategy Lazarus and Launier (1978) describe are: information seeking, direct action, inhibition of action, and intrapsychic processes. Each mode, with the possible exception of the last, can serve both instrumental and palliative functions. Increasing one's knowledge about the problem situation can aid in decision making and the selection of coping strategies. It can also remove the threat by enabling a reappraisal of the situation as irrelevant or benign and can also serve the palliative function of 'making the person feel better, by rationalizing, or bolstering a past decision' (Lazarus, 1982, p 176). Direct action is really a self-explanatory mode of coping. Sometimes, however, action can be impulsive but detrimental. Controlling one's aggressive impulses is a good example of the value of 'inhibition of action'. Intrapsychic modes of coping include all the things people say to themselves in an attempt to reduce the emotional impact of a problem situation. The classical psychoanalytic defence mechanisms of denial, avoidance, reaction formation, projection and repression, etc., are all examples of intrapsychic coping strategies.

Coping resources, Lazarus stresses, are quite distinct and far more stable than the actual strategies used. They are important for the coping process as they provide a basis for both appraisal and coping action. Folkman et al (1979) suggests there are at least five main types or categories of coping resource: (1) health/energy/moral; (2) problem solving skills; (3) utilitarian resources (e.g. money, social agencies); (4) general and specific beliefs; and (5) social networks. The influence of the first two coping resources on primary and secondary appraisal and the coping process is quite self evident and that of the third and fifth has already been discussed. General and specific beliefs are likely to stem from both socialization and past experience. A belief that is likely to be particularly important in determining coping behaviour is the belief in self efficacy or control. Clearly if one believes one has no control over a situation then attempts at instrumental control will be reduced or even waived (Folkman and Lazarus, 1980) and emotional-focused coping increased. Perceived control will also affect primary appraisal and, hence, the need for emotional-focused coping. The importance of perceptions of control in the aetiology of psychological distress is considered below.

Research on Coping In RA

With the exception of one study (Felton and Revenson, 1984 - reviewed in the section on knowledge and adjustment below) there does not appear to have been any systematic investigations of coping in RAs. However, there have been some attempts to teach coping strategies such as biofeedback (Denver et al, 1979), relaxation (Achterberg et al, 1981), stress innoculation (Randich, 1982), and exercises (Achterberg et al, 1981) to RAs (see Anderson et al, 1985, for a review). Unfortunately, the extent to which these strategies helped relieve psychological distress is not reported, although typically, they did decrease patients reports of pain and increase functional capacity.

CONTROL

Experimental work with both humans and animals indicates that the perception of control influences emotional reactions to stressors (see Abramson and Seligman, 1978; Thompson, 1981; Langer, 1983; for reviews of this evidence).

Learned Helplessness Theory

The most important theoretical formulation linking control and psychological distress is Learned Helplessness (LH) Theory (Seligman, 1975).

Seligman proposed that depressive affect, along with associated cognitive and motivational deficits, could result from a lack of control over the environment, or non-contingent reinforcement. According to Seligman, the initial response to a stressful situation is anxiety, but this is replaced by depression if the person comes to believe that control is unattainable. Much experimental evidence supports this theory (e.g. Hiroto, 1974; Hiroto and Seligman, 1975; Klein and Seligman, 1976). Hiroto (1974), for example, found previous exposure to uncontrollable noise led to reduced attempts after control when control was possible (motivational deficit), it also made it difficult for subjects to recognise contingency in later trials (cognitive deficit), and the emotional response accompanying these deficits was described as depressive in nature.

It has been suggested, however, that LH theory is too simplistic to account for human helplessness and a reformulation has been developed (Abramson and Seligman, 1978). The main refinement to the original model is the distinction of three orthogonal dimensions of helplessness: universal-personal, stable-unstable, and global-specific. Personal (internal) helplessness is when a person's belief in non-contingency is founded on a belief in personal ineffectualness and a belief that others in the same situation are not helpless, while universal (external) helplessness entails the belief that non-contingency is externally caused and that everyone is helpless. The dimension of stability reflects the extent to which feelings of helplessness are transient or chronic. Finally, feelings of helplessness may be confined to specific situations or they may be evident in most or all situations.

This reformulation is better able to account for the human evidence, for example, the finding of Douglas and Anisman (1975) that task complexity influenced whether failure at a given task affected later cognitive performance - failure of the simple task produced a cognitive deficit, while failure of the complex task did not. In terms of the reformulated model of LH this is because failure of a complex task can be attributed to the task difficulty (i.e. an external attribution can be made) while failure at the simple task can only be attributed to personal inadequacy (i.e. an internal attribution).

According to the original model non-contingency produced all three types of deficit - i.e. affective, motivational, and cognitive. In the reformulation depressed affect is attributed to the expectation that bad outcomes will occur or that good ones will not. This modification was suggested by negative evidence - the finding that positive life events are not associated with psychological disorder. However, there is evidence to suggest an attributional bias - a tendency to attribute success to ourselves and failure to chance (Langer, 1983) - and this bias might equally explain the above result.

The inadequacy of the original model highlights the problems of extrapolating from animal experiments. Seligman's early animal experimental work (e.g. Seligman and Maier, 1967) was not only barbaric but also futile and misleading. It was not until the model was tested on humans that its shortcomings were brought to light.

<u>Social Learning theory and the Locus of Control Concept</u>

A fairly similar conceptualization of control is evident in Social Learning Theory (e.g. Rotter, 1982). Basically, this theory suggests behaviour, or behaviour potential, will occur if the perpetrator believes the behaviour will produce a certain outcome that is valued. Individuals are assumed to differ in terms of their generalized expectancies about the source, or locus, of control over events.

Early measures of the locus of control concept (Rotter, 1966) distinguished just one dimension of locus of control, internal-external. High scorers on this scale (internals) tend to attribute control over events to themselves while low scorers (externals) believe events are controlled by external forces such as powerful others and chance. More recently some scales have been developed which distinguish beliefs in powerful others from beliefs in chance (Levenson, 1973) - a distinction similar to that drawn between universal and personal helplessness in the revised LH Theory. There has also been a trend to develop more reinforcer-specific locus of control scales. Various questionnaires have been developed to assess beliefs about sources of control over particular aspects of health such as weight loss (Saltzer, 1979) and pain (Skevington, in press), but most widely used in the domain of health research is the Health Locus of Control Scale (HLC; Wallston et al, 1976) and the Multidimensional Health Locus of Control Scale (MHLC; Wallston et al, 1978), both of which assess beliefs about health in general as opposed to specific health issues. The difference between these two questionnaires lies in the fact that the latter comprises three subscales - 'internality' (IHLC), 'powerful others' (PHLC), and 'chance' (CHLC) - while the former is unidimensional.

Researchers have most frequently looked for an association between beliefs in control and health behaviour (Ell, 1986). Evidence relating beliefs about control over physical illness with psychological adjustment in the physically ill is rather sparse and mainly comprises descriptive studies. However, internality, assessed by the HLC scale, has been found to be positively associated with life satisfaction and the will to live amongst geriatric pacemaker patients (Brown et al, 1981); past and future expectations of life satisfaction amongst chronic dialysis patients (Hatz, 1978); presurgical anxiety (Lowery et al, 1975); and post-surgical duration of hospitalization and use of analgesics (Clum et al, 1979); while CHLC has been reported as correlating significantly and positively with depression among general medical patients (Donham et al, 1983), epileptics (DeVellis et al, 1980,) and cancer patients undergoing chemotherapy (reported in Wallson and Wallston, 1982). Depression has also been reported as correlating positively with PHLC but to a lesser extent than with CHLC (DeVellis et al, 1980,).

One study has examined the relationship of beliefs in control and psychological distress in a sample of RAs. Felton and Revenson (1984) report that patients' (hypertensives, diabetics, RAs and cancer patients) rating of the controllability of their illness explained significant proportions of 'illness acceptance' variance even after the effects of diagnosis was removed.

The fairly consistent association of depression with chance beliefs is in line with the LH Theory of depression. Notably, however, only one of the studies mentioned above found an association of PHLC and depression, and internal locus of control has been found to be positively associated with both measures of adjustment (e.g. life satisfaction) and psychological distress (e.g. anxiety). Possibly understanding of adjustment to illness might be advanced by considering the pattern of scores on the MHLC scales. Wallston and Wallston (1982) present a typology of health locus of control beliefs based on whether an individual scores relatively high or low on each of the three dimensions of locus of control distinguished in the MHLC scale.

Given the finding by Langer (1975, 1977) that a perception of control may be adaptive even in the absence of objective control, the presenters of this typology (Wallston and Wallston, 1982) suggest the most adaptive pattern of beliefs in illness may be what they call 'type V' ('believers in control' - high scorers on both PHLC and IHLC) or possibly type VII (high scorers on all three scales). In this latter instance it is argued that a belief in chance, in addition to beliefs in powerful others and personal control, may be beneficial in so much as it '.. provide(s) a convenient rationalization for those instances where one's best shot and the best efforts of others have all come to naught' (p 71, Wallston and Wallston, 1982).

Only one study has examined the value of this typology in predicting psychological adjustment in illness, and surprisingly it was conducted with a sample of RAs (Roskam, 1985). This researcher reports that, among Ss reporting a high frequency of flare-ups, 'believers in control' (type V) were found to have the lowest levels of depression.

ILLNESS KNOWLEDGE

The importance of knowledge or information seeking as a coping strategy has already been discussed briefly during a consideration of Lazarus and colleagues' model of coping. To reiterate, Lazarus suggests three main functions of information: (1) aids decision making and selection of coping strategies; (2) removes or reduces threat by enabling a reappraisal of the situation as more benign than initially thought and; (3) rationalizes or supports a past decision.

Ley (1982) with specific reference to the role of information in affecting emotional responses to medical treatment and investigatory procedures suggests four functions of information: (1) enables covert rehearsal, and thus, habituation prior to the experience; (2) provision of labels for experiences and sensations which would otherwise be unlabelled and thus, possibly, interpreted as negative affect; (3) increasing feelings of control; and (4) stimulation of moderate fear and realistic expectations.

Evidence for the occurrence of these hypothesized functions of information in coping with physical illness is rather limited and that there is, mainly concerned with rather short lived procedures, which Ss have not previously experienced, such as surgery (see Ley, 1982; and Mathews and Ridgeway, 1984; for reviews). Typically, such studies have assessed the impact of various pre-operative interventions, among them various informational manipulations, on recovery; 'mood' or psychological adjustment is sometimes considered as one of several dependent variables. Unfortunately, from the point of view of looking at the effect of information on adjustment, the majority of studies are methodologically flawed. Often there have been no controls for attention and another common fault is the confounding of different types of intervention. Mathews and Ridgeway (1984), however, report five controlled studies looking at post-operative mood following an unconfounded, pre-operative, informational, intervention - none found any affect of information on post-operative mood. Furthermore, studies contrasting an informational intervention with other types of intervention (behavioural instructions, cognitive coping strategies, discussion of worries, etc.) typically report that information is less beneficial with regards to other criteria of recovery (e.g. length of hospitalization; analgesic use) (see Mathews and Ridgeway, 1984).

The effect of the content of the informational intervention has also received a little attention. Johnson et al (1978) compared procedural and sensation information in cholecystectomy and hernia surgical patients. While it appears neither intervention had any affect on post-operative mood, sensation information was associated with a shorter duration of hospitalization, while procedural information was not associated with any outcome measure.

Ley's (1982a) last function of information (see above) is based on the idea of 'emotional inoculation' (Janis, 1958), which suggests that ".. preparatory communications are effective when they arouse a moderate level of anticipatory fear, which leads to the constructive 'work of worry', that is mentally rehearsing the impending threats and developing realistic, self delivered reassurances that prevent subsequent emotional shocks .." (p197; Langer, 1983). More recently, however, research has emphasised the advantages of denial (which typically is seen as the antithesis of realism) in coping with illness (Meyerwitz, 1980, 1983; Levine and Zigler, 1975; Beisser, 1979; Stourkes, 1982) and several studies have failed to find the hypothesized curvilinear relationship between pre-operative fear and post-operative recovery (Levy and McGee, 1975; Sime, 1976; Ley, 1977; Leventhal et al, 1979).

For at least two reasons information seeking would seem to be a particularly valuable coping strategy in RA.

First, in the absence of information or knowledge people make estimates about probability utilizing a number of heuristics (Tversky and Kahneman, 1977). Of relevance to this discussion is the heuristic of 'availability', which refers to the ease with which instances of the event in question can be brought to mind. Because the ease with which it is possible to recall instances of an event is affected by factors other than actual frequency, this heuristic leads to certain biases. In any illness the worst cases tend to be more visible and, hence, memorable, but in RA they are perhaps more noticeable and identifiable than in many other illnesses due to the occurrence of characteristic deformities and disability. This visibility and identifiability of the worst cases is likely to make most people overestimate the negative effects of RA, additionally, patients attending a rheumatology clinic are actually likely to be disproportionately exposed to the more severe cases of RA, as these are the patients who will most likely be frequent and repeated attenders at the clinic. Hence, one would anticipate that patients without the benefit of accurate information regarding prognosis will tend to overestimate the risks.

Secondly, the nature of the condition - high, apparently non-contingent, intrapersonal variability is more characteristic of RA than of many other conditions - is likely to make sufferers particularly vulnerable to feelings of hopelessness and helplessness. Consequently the hypothesis that knowledge produces feelings of control would seem particularly relevant. Advising patients that pain variability does not mean control is unattainable or that treatments are not working may reinstate hope and feelings of control to some extent.

Additionally, patients with RA often feel a degree of guilt or self blame for their condition and are perhaps particularly likely to feel unattractive and prematurely old because of their illness (Rogers et al, 1982). Again it seems likely that information may allay some of these misgivings

Although there have been many knowledge intervention studies with RAs (see for example, Lorig et al, 1984, 1985b; Vignos et al, 1976; Schwartz et al, 1978) very few have assessed psychological adjustment as a dependent variable and those that have are, typically, limited and methodologically unsound. None the less, a number of studies have reported a positive effect of knowledge. Wetsone et al (1982), looking at the effects of a computer based education program for RAs, reports that patients in the experimental group showed a significantly 'improved outlook on life' and were 'more optimistic about the prognosis of their disease' relative to controls. Unfortunately details are not given regarding the assessment of knowledge or 'attitudes', or regarding the control conditions, and the entire sample, including experimental and control groups comprised just 36 Ss. Kaye and Hammond (1978) report that 54% of their sample of 48 RAs reported changes in feelings ('predominantly positive') regarding their disease and 42% reported positive changes in feelings regarding themselves following an information intervention. Again, however, the validity and reliability of these assessments is not established and in this study there was no control group. Finally, one study provides rather ambiguous support for the importance of illness knowledge in psychological adjustment. Kaplan and Kozin (1981) compared an education only intervention with an education plus counselling intervention (experimental group). While they found no improvement in self-esteem in either group, depression (assessed by the SDS) was decreased in the experimental group but only after the educational component of the program.

The value of information seeking as a coping strategy was evaluated in four categories of chronically ill patients (hypertensives, diabetics, RAs, and cancer patients) which the authors (Felton and Revenson, 1984) suggest are distinguished in terms of disease controllability (RA and cancer being least and hypertension most controllable). Information seeking was measured by a five item scale which assessed the extent to which patients: looked up medical information; read books or magazines or watched TV programs about their illness; found several different solutions to a problem; asked someone other than a physician for advice; and made a plan of action and followed it. Regardless of illness category, information seeking was associated with decreased negative affect. A time-lag analysis supported a direction of causality such that coping strategy affected adjustment. Felton and Revenson suggest several explanations for the constructive effects of information seeking, including the suggestions that: symptoms are made more meaningful; the well-informed are more likely to engage in appropriate health practices; information serves a palliative function, acting as an 'emotional-focused attention deployment strategy'; and the suggestion that 'information seeking may reflect the kind of optimistic mental framework that reinforces the idea that the information obtained will be useful ' (p 351).

Contradictory evidence is provided by a study by Parker and colleagues (1984) who reported that their educational intervention was not related to changes in BDI scores but was associated with increased reports of pain - a finding opposite to that of Lorig and colleagues (Lorig, 1984; Lorig et al, 1984, 1985). In both the control and experimental groups, however, decreases in depression were associated with medical interventions. Yet again, however, the S sample was very small (N=22) and in this instance comprised solely of men, and although there was a control group there was no control for attention.

One other study (N=127) reports the lack of a significant correlation between valid and reliable measures of knowledge and psychological adjustment in RAs (Lorish et al, 1985).

The relationship of different types of knowledge with adjustment in RA does not appear to have undergone investigation .

POSITIVE REACTIONS TO ILLNESS

So far this review has concentrated on negative reactions to illness; this very much reflects the bias of the research literature. However, a few people have described positive changes in psychosocial functioning following a major adverse health event. Lipowski (1970), talking about 'illness as value' says,

> 'One thing seems beyond question; the experience of illness may enhance the intensity and depth of the experience of living and this can be reflected in thought, feeling and action. Is there a higher mode of coping available to man?' (p 100)

He points to lives of famous men - including Bach, Beethoven and Proust - as examples of this superior mode of coping.

Similarly, White and Liddon (1972), describing the psychological reactions of survivors of cardiac arrest, note that five of the 10 patients studied experienced what they describe as a 'transcendental redirection'. In three cases this took the form of a 'religious conversion' or experience while in the two other instances the experience is more aptly describe as 'philosophical readjustment'. The case study of a patient in this latter category is most illuminating:

> 'Prior to the arrest ... She claimed that she had had little regard for her fellow man and had been occupied mainly with material concerns ... During her stay in the intensive care unit she did much thinking about the nature of life and contemplated changing her outlook. She stated that life had more to offer than she had realized, and she felt she had spent too much of her life worrying about small, insignificant details.' (p 223)

Finally, Matson and Brooks (1977) report that for some of the patients in their sample 'multiple sclerosis had afforded then time to get in touch with the more essential values in life ... turning the disease into a positive force' (p 248). Again, in some cases, Matson notes this orientation was associated with religious faith which, incidentally, was the most prevalent coping strategy mentioned in answer to the question 'what has most helped you to cope?'

To date, however, investigations of this positive reaction to illness have been subjective and anecdotal, and the relationship of this response to other psychological and disease related variables has not been investigated.

CHAPTER 3

COMPLIANCE WITH MEDICAL ADVICE

INCIDENCE OF NON-COMPLIANCE

It has been said that 'the desire to take medicine is perhaps the greatest feature which distinguishes man from animals' (Osler, quoted in Cushing, 1925). However, Podell (1975) concludes that on average physicians' instructions are followed correctly by only one third of all patients. Ley (1979a) reviews 49 studies of medication compliance levels for four different types of medication (T.B. drugs; antibiotics; antacids and iron etc.; and psychotropic drugs) and reports non-compliance levels ranging from 8-92%, with the average level of non-compliance being 42.5%. Neither is this rather high level of non-compliance accounted for by the psychiatric patients - mean non-compliance with psychotropic drugs across the nine relevant studies was only 39%.

Compliance with other forms of medical advice is no greater than that for medication. Becker and Rosenstock (1984), in a review of the literature, report that medical appointments are unattended 20-50% of the time, and that smoking cessation programs are considered to be 'unusually effective' if only a third of clients are still smoking less than originally after six months. Ley (1979a) reports non-compliance levels between 20 and 84% across 11 studies of compliance with diet advice.

Having scoured the literature between 1962 and 1982 for relevant papers, Belcon et al (1984) cites 19 studies which report compliance levels with various aspects of medical advice among RAs. Compliance with prescribed drug regimens, across the eight relevant studies, ranged from 16 to 84%. For physiotherapy the range of compliance levels was from 39 to 65%, while splints were used as intended in 25 to 65% of cases.

Compliance is generally considered to be objectively rational, but if this is so, why are people non-compliant? The psychological literature on this topic is overwhelmingly vast (although, notably, there has not been that much relevant research on compliance in RA), confusing and marked by inconsistent findings.

PROBLEMS WITH COMPLIANCE RESEARCH

Most of the research conducted on the issue of compliance has been atheoretical. This has resulted in a rather amorphous literature. Additionally, a number of unresolved methodological issues make drawing comparisons across studies difficult and may account for the seeming contradictions among studies.

(1) Lack of an Agreed Definition of Compliance

Haynes et al (1979) defines compliance as, '.. the extent to which a person's behaviour ... coincides with medical or health advice.' Unfortunately, different researchers have tended to define, or at least, operationalize, compliance differently (Ley, 1979a; Becker and Rosenstock, 1984). Some adopt an 'all or nothing' approach, where any deviation from the regimen is deemed non-compliance. At the other end of the scale, some researchers have only classed patients as non-compliant where compliance is below the level necessary for therapeutic effect or where the regimen is not adhered to at all. Others simply divide patients at the median into compliant and non-compliant groups, and some divide patients on seemingly arbitrary grounds or in terms of some criteria of compliance they feel is significant. Sometimes patients who do follow the prescribed regimen but also take other drugs, not prescribed by their doctors, or visit unorthodox practitioners, are considered non-compliant (e.g. Hulka et al, 1975).

(2) Heterogeneity of Assessment Methods

Where the behaviour in question is readily observable and recorded, such as follow-up and referral appointment keeping, uptake of vaccinations or screening, then assessment is, clearly, straightforward. Typically, however, it is not.

A variety of methods of assessment have been used, including: self-report (Ley, 1983; Kincey, 1975; Ferguson and Boyle, 1979); pill counts (Ley et al, 1975; Sacket et al, 1975; Nugent et al, 1965; Joyce, 1962; Wasner et al, 1981; Mason et al, 1967); blood and urine assays of drug metabolites (Joyce, 1962; Ferguson and Boyle, 1979); clinicians' judgements (Francis et al, 1969; De Wet and Hollinshead, 1980; Geersten et al, 1973); and outcome (Ley et al, 1974). Some studies have reported high intercorrelations between the different methods of assessment (e.g. Feinstein et al, 1959; Francis et al, 1969; Becker et al, 1972, 1978) -

although, Becker and Rosenstock (1984) suggest this may reflect patient awareness that their compliance is being monitored and double checked. Other studies have found substantial differences in compliance rates depending on the method of assessment. Gordis et al (1969), for example, found that rates of non-compliance were greatest using blood and urine assays, followed by pill counts and then self-report.

What is certain is that no method of assessment is unproblematical. Almost certainly the most unreliable and invalid are outcome measures and clinical assessments (which, in fact, are likely to be based largely on outcome). The relationship between compliance and outcome is far from perfect; apart from anything else, there are good theoretical reasons for expecting the worst cases to be most compliant. Self-report is also, typically, considered fairly low down on the list of good methods, but this perhaps reflects the behavioural researchers dislike of phenomenological data and all things kin, as, in fact, the alternative methods are just as problematical. Pill counts are just as subject to deception on the part of the patient as self-report, additionally, accidental loss of tablets or unreported or unremembered sharing or decanting of medication may make this method even more unreliable. The validity of blood and urine assays - often assumed to be the most reliable and valid measures - is also questionable, due to intra and inter-individual differences in drug metabolism. This method is also invasive and expensive.

(3) Dimensions of Health Behaviour

The behaviours actually studied are, like the methods of assessment, pretty diverse. The possibility that different sets of determinants are needed to understand different types of compliant behaviour has led to some attempts to distinguish subcategories of health behaviour.

In terms of literature reviews of the area (e.g. Becker and Rosenstock, 1984) and research papers, the most widely used categorization of health behaviours is that proposed by Kasl and Cobb (1966) - based on the Parsonian (1951) formulation of the 'sick role' - which distinguishes: (a) preventive health behaviour (PHB) - behaviour undertaken to prevent disease or detect it in its asymptomatic state by people who believe themselves to be healthy; (b) illness behaviour - behaviour undertaken by people who feel ill for the purpose of defining their state of health and obtaining a remedy; and (c) sick role behaviour - behaviour undertaken by the individual who is already labelled ill for the purpose of getting well.

Refinements to this tripartite distinction of health, illness and sick role behaviours have been proposed. Kasl (1974) for example, suggests an additional classification of the 'at-risk role' in particular to account for some of the behaviours observable in chronic illness; behaviours such as staying in treatment to prevent deterioration rather than produce a cure, or staying in treatment when well because of the knowledge that one or more risk factors are present (e.g. as in hypertension). He has also proposed a distinction between screening and other types of PHB (e.g. antenatal visits, vaccinations etc.). The former, he suggests, is more akin to illness behaviour, being motivated by symptoms the 'patient' does not acknowledge.

Kasl (1974) has also suggested a general criterion for classifying health behaviours, namely, their consequences, whether negative, neutral or positive. Thus, for example, screening, Kasl suggests, has neutral (no disease detected) and negative (disease detected) consequences, while vaccinations have positive (prevent infection) and neutral (no effect) consequences. In reality, however, this approach is far too simplistic; most health behaviours, if not all, can be seen to carry the possibility of all three outcomes. Vaccinations, for example, have an incidence of serious side-effects as do most treatments.

The question of the validity of these various classifications appears to have undergone very little research but what evidence there is suggests they are inadequate. Specific behaviours, even within the various subcategories, do not appear to be related. With regard to sick role behaviour, Berkowitz et al (1963), for example, found that appointment keeping was unrelated to medication adherence. Ferguson and Boyle (1979) report that RA patients were 'selectively' non-compliant, compliance with aspirin or exercise advice being unrelated to compliance with other aspects of the regimen. Similarly, Schafer et al (1983) report that, among their sample of diabetics, adherence to one aspect of the regimen was not associated with adherence to other aspects of the regimen. PHBs also tend to be largely uncorrelated (e.g. Kristiansen, 1984).

The only factor analytic studies of health behaviour appear to have been restricted to a consideration of PHBs (see Kristiansen, 1984, for a review of such studies). Langlie (1979), for example, concludes that there are two dimensions of PHB: 'direct risk' behaviours (e.g. not smoking or drinking and driving) and 'indirect risk' behaviours (e.g. immunization, check-ups, seat-belt use). Others, however, suggest the need for further differentiation (e.g. Harris and Guton, 1979; Kristiansen, 1984). Kristiansen, for example, in an analysis of some 148 PHBs, concludes that the vast majority of variance is unique! Clearly, the results of those studies which have simply lumped together different health behaviours in a scale, without any concern for underlying factor structure (e.g. Butler, 1980; DeVellis et al, 1980b), are of questionable validity.

FACTORS ASSOCIATED WITH COMPLIANCE

A lack of theory has resulted in what has been termed 'shot-gun' research (Becker and Maiman, 1975) into the issue of compliance and there is a consequent wealth of research relating a wealth of different variables to compliance. Clearly, in a review of this nature, or, indeed, in any review of the compliance literature, there is a need for selectivity. In this review the relationship of compliance with four main types or categories of variable will be considered, namely: health beliefs, illness knowledge, health locus of control, and the doctor-patient relationship. These are selected because they represent the most theoretical and interesting approaches to the issue and subsume many of the more idiosyncratic variables.

HEALTH BELIEFS

The health belief model (HBM), attributed to Rosenstock (1966), was first developed to explain 'PHB' but has since been extended to explain 'sick role' and 'illness' behaviour.

Basically, the HBM is a form of value-expectancy model. Very similar models have been developed by others interested in explaining behaviour (e.g. Tolman, 1955; Rotter, 1954; Edwards, 1954; Atkinson, 1957, Fishbein and Ajzen, 1975). Specifically, the HBM states that health behaviour is determined by the relative weight and interaction of three factors. As Becker and Rosenstock (1984) describe them:

(1) the individual's subjective state of readiness to take action, which is determined by both the person's perceived susceptibility to the particular illness and by his or her perceptions of the probable severity of the physical and social consequences of contracting the disease;

(2) the individual's evaluation of the advocated health behaviour, in terms of its feasibility and efficaciousness (i.e. an estimate of the action's potential benefits in reducing susceptibility and/or severity), weighed against perceptions of physical, psychological, financial, and other costs or barriers involved in the proposed action; and

(3) a cue to action must occur to trigger the appropriate health behaviour; this stimulus can be either internal (e.g. the perception of symptoms) or external (e.g. interpersonal interactions, mass media communications. (p 180. Reprinted by permission of Academic Press)

Extension of the model by Becker (1976) to include 'modifying factors' such as 'diverse demographic, personal, structural and social factors', arguably, enables the model to incorporate most of the data in the field. These modifying factors are not considered to be direct causes of health behaviour, but rather are assumed to exert their influence via the other components of the model (Becker and Rosenstock, 1984). The explanatory power of the extended model is impressive, but, arguably, at a cost of being practically untestable.

Quite a few studies have examined the relationship of one or more HBM variables with compliance - often, in fact, without acknowledging the HBM - (see Becker and Rosenstock, 1984; Ley, 1979; Haynes and Sackett, 1977, for reviews), and the weight of evidence suggests that they are fairly consistent predictors of health behaviour of all types. Prospective studies (see Becker and Rosenstock, 1984, for a review), although a little scarce, also support the direction of causality implied by the model. However, the possibility, suggested by some (e.g. Taylor, 1979), that health beliefs represent adhoc rationalizations for behaviour is consistent with Cognitive Dissonance theory (Festinger, 1957) and a substantial body of evidence looking at the development of attitudes or beliefs about other issues (see Eiser, 1980, for a review of some of this evidence), and cannot be ruled out.

Only three studies have assessed the relationship of any of the HBM variables and compliance in RAs and surprisingly the weight of evidence here does not support the model. However, all three studies are methodologically flawed.

Carpenter and Davis (1976) assessed patients beliefs about the severity of their arthritis and their perception of the perceived benefits of the prescribed exercise regimen and report that neither variable was associated with compliance. However, these researchers do not make explicit their operationalization of compliance. Furthermore, they give no information about the validity and reliability of their perception of arthritis severity scale and the assessment of patients' perceptions of treatment benefits was rather insensitive (one yes/no response item).

Ferguson and Bole (1979) report that in their cross-sectional study of 40 RAs a belief in the benefit of treatment was the only significant predictor of compliance, but even this only predicted compliance with aspirin and not with splints. Again, however, belief in benefit was assessed by a single yes/no question per treatment and their definition of non-compliance was seemingly arbitrary. Patients who reported 'often' not taking their aspirin or who wore their splints less than three times a week were deemed non-compliant.

Finally, Geersten et al (1973), in a particularly problematic study, failed to find a significant difference in level of compliance among RA patients experiencing pain or discomfort as a result of treatment and those who did not experience these side-effects. However, patients who thought the crippling effects of arthritis were inevitable or who felt treatment would be unsuccessful were significantly less compliant, as were patients who were kept waiting a long time when they visited the clinic or expressed irritation over being kept waiting. In this study, however, patients were classified as 'full' or 'partial' compliers on the basis of whether the physician thought they were taking their medications or not and attending the clinic as often as advised; and different aspects of the regimen were not distinguished.

KNOWLEDGE

Several researchers have reported that their educational intervention led to an increase in RAs' self care behaviours (Wetstone, 1982; Lorig et al, 1984; Lorig, 1985b; Knudson et al, 1981; Kaye and Hammond, 1978). Unfortunately, it is not made clear in these studies to what extent this increase represents an increase in compliance, as to what extent patients were aware of these behaviours or had been instructed to do them prior to the intervention is not reported. One study (Carpenter and Davis, 1976) of RAs reports a tendency (non-significant) for the less well informed to be most compliant. However, both the measures of understanding and compliance are problematical in this study. Understanding was judged simply as 'poor' or 'good' by a social worker and 'general compliance' was judged by the clinician.

Studies looking at non-RA patients (see Ley, 1982a, for a comprehensive review) have found both a positive association of these two variables and no association. A simple negative relationship between knowledge and compliance has not been reported in the literature, although, Cromwell and Levenkron (1984) report an interaction of knowledge with coping style. Coronary patients who were coping by denying or repression were less co-operative with nurses if they were in the 'information condition', while 'sensitizers' benefitted from the provision of information.

The inconsistency of findings in the literature has led some reviewers (e.g. Jenny, 1983; Becker and Rosenstock, 1984) to be rather dismissive of the importance of knowledge in predicting compliance, but this is really a little premature. In addition to the methodological problems discussed above, there are a number of other possible reasons why patient knowledge and compliance might not always seem to be related.

First, some reviewers of the area are dismissing the hypothesis without a proper consideration of the evidence. Morris and Halperin (1979), for example, review the evidence relating the provision of written information with compliance and report that while information improved short-term compliance in six out of seven studies, it improved long-term compliance in only six out of 11 studies. Ley (1982), however, in a re-examination of these studies, reports that in only five did an analysis of knowledge levels show that the experimental group actually had more knowledge than the control group, and of these five, four reported the experimental group to be more compliant.

Secondly, studies which fail to report an association of knowledge and compliance have often used very general measures of patient knowledge, or in the case of intervention studies (e.g. Sackett et al, 1975; Gross and Brandt, 1981; Kirscht and Rosenstock, 1979) given patients fairly non-specific and general information regarding their illness. Where knowledge is more specifically relevant to the regimen then compliance has been reported as being strongly related to knowledge (e.g. Svarstad, 1974) and similarly, informational interventions which provide patients with more specific information are generally successful in increasing compliance levels (e.g. McKenney et al, 1973).

Thirdly, non-compliance is unlikely to be determined by a single key variable. As with most behaviours it is likely to be multi-determined and the predictive weight of any particular independent variable is likely to vary from both person to person and treatment to treatment. The failure of some studies to find an association between knowledge and compliance may simply reflect the fact that for the particular sample of patients or treatment regimen involved, or indeed, the interaction of these two, knowledge is of little importance in determining compliance.

A Typology of Non-Compliance

Ley (1979a, 1982a) has proposed a 2x2 classification, or typology, of non-compliance in terms of both motivation and knowledge (see Fig. 3.1).

Figure 3.1

Types of non-compliance and suggested remedial action

(Ley, 1982a, p 361. Reprinted by permission of John Wiley and Sons, Ltd.)

Types of Non-Compliance	Knowledge and Comprehension	
	Adequate	Inadequate
Intentional	persuasive techniques	information
Unintentional	aids to memory	information

According to Ley the success of informational interventions in increasing compliance will depend on the proportion of patients in each category; information can only possibly lead to increased compliance (but even then does not necessarily do so) if the patient is initially inadequately informed.

In discussing his typology, Ley is rather evasive with regards to the question of what it is to be 'adequately informed', although, his distinction of 'inadequately informed unintentional non-compliers' (patients who think they are being compliant but simply do not know what to do) and 'inadequately informed intentional non-compliers' perhaps suggests it involves more than basic knowledge about the regimen, such as what to do and how to do it. In a previous section of his review on 'Giving Information to Patients', Ley (1982a), reviews various criteria for deciding what information should be given and it seems likely that his criterion of 'rationality' would distinguish the 'inadequately informed' from the 'adequately informed'. According to this criteria patients should be given enough information to make rational decisions about treatment. Specifically, as Ley (1982a) puts it, knowledge regarding:

'(1) the probabilities of improvement, no improvement and of deterioration both with and without treatment; and

(2) the nature and probabilities of occurrence of side-effects and adverse reactions.' (p 350).

In terms of the HBM this represents information about the 'costs' and 'benefits' of treatment. The extent to which providing patients with this information leads to increased compliance is likely to depend on their ability to understand and remember this information (Ley et al, 1975; Ley, 1977) - i.e. their actual knowledge or beliefs - and on their initial beliefs. Compliance will increase to the extent that information increases patients' perceptions of the 'net benefit' of treatment.

<u>Path by Which Knowledge Affects Compliance</u>

Ley (1982a, 1985) suggests two routes, a direct and an indirect route, for the influence of knowledge on compliance (see Fig. 3.2).

Figure 3.2

Routes via which knowledge may affect compliance - Ley's 'cognitive model'

(Ley, 1982, p 360. Reprinted by permission of John Wiley and Sons, Ltd.)

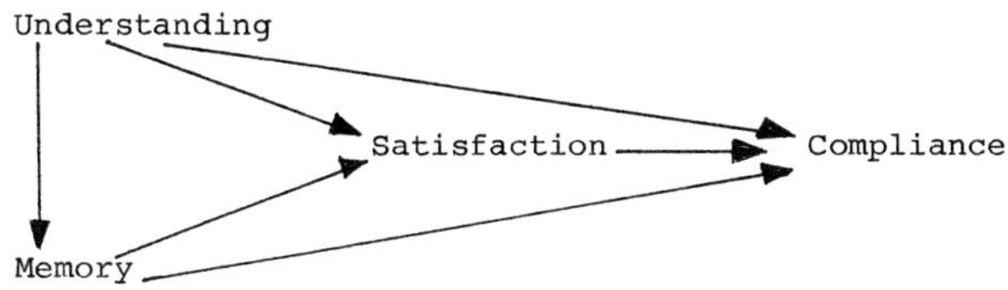

Patient satisfaction is one of the few variables which has been found to be fairly consistently related to patient compliance (Ley, 1982a, 1985; Haynes, 1976). Unfortunately, Ley does not suggest how patient satisfaction actually influences compliance. Practically it seems it may be synonymous with the HBM concept of 'net benefit'. In terms of its operationalization, satisfaction has been defined as either satisfaction with information or communications (e.g. Ley and Spelman, 1967; Ley et al, 1976a, 1976b), or more generally as satisfaction with the consultation as a whole (e.g. Bertakis, 1977; Francis et al, 1969; Brody, 1980). General satisfaction is likely to reflect satisfaction with: information; the doctor-patient relationship; treatment; and a few miscellaneous things such as waiting time and conditions, and convenience of attendance. All of these can be seen to contribute to patients' perceptions of the 'net benefit' of compliance.

THE DOCTOR-PATIENT RELATIONSHIP

The quality of the doctor-patient relationship, it has been claimed, and indeed, evidence supports the idea, is an important determinant of patient compliance (e.g. Jenny, 1983; Becker and Rosenstock, 1984; Hauser, 1981; Geersten et al, 1973). Two interrelated aspects of doctor-patient communication are generally distinguished (e.g. Hauser, 1981): the communication of information, and the communication of affect. Both are likely to affect compliance.

Communication of Information

The importance of the provision to the patient of understandable and recallable information has already been discussed in this review. Equally important is the provision of information by the patient. First, if the doctor is to be effective in providing information for the patient (s)he must know what to provide and this information is most accurately obtained from the patient. Secondly, unless the doctor is, and is seen to be, fully cognizant with the problem, (s)he is unlikely to prescribe correct or acceptable treatment, and patients are likely to question the accuracy of their diagnosis and the appropriateness of the prescribed treatment, and, hence, the value of compliance. Evidence that doctors often do miss or ignore patients' major symptoms (Maguire and Rutter, 1976) suggests that this factor may be an important contributor to non-compliance. Just why communication of information is so poor in the doctor-patient relationship is another issue and one dealt with later in this chapter.

Communication of Affect

The importance of the affective component of the doctor-patient relationship in predicting compliance is illustrated in a study by Korsh and Negrete (1972) in which it was found that the proportion of 'negative affect' (disagreements, tension, antagonism) expressed in the consultation was inversely related to 'maternal compliance' (i.e. the extent mothers followed or enforced treatment recommendations for their children). The expression of 'positive affect' by the doctor was associated with increased compliance and satisfaction.

Tentative evidence that the affective component of the relationship may actually be more important than the information component in predicting compliance is provided in a study by Geersten et al (1973), which, incidentally, appears to be the only study which has addressed the question of the relationship between the doctor-patient relationship and compliance in RA. In this study three aspects of the doctor-patient relationship were assessed: doctor to patient communication; patient to doctor communication; and the 'nature of the relationship', whether 'personal' or 'business-like'. The latter variable was the only one significantly associated with compliance - 'full compliers' were more likely to experience a 'personal' relationship than 'partial compliers'. Unfortunately, the validity of this research is questionable as the assessment of both independent and dependent variables is methodologically dubious. Patients were simply designated as 'full' or 'partial compliers' on the basis of physicians' ratings and details of the development, content, validity and reliability of the scales designed to detect difficulties in communication, and of the assessment of the 'nature of the relationship' are not given.

There are a number of possible routes via which the affective component of the doctor-patient relationship might affect compliance. First, where the tone of the relationship is relaxed and open, communication is likely to be better. Secondly, if the doctor appears kindly and concerned the patient is more likely to feel assured that he will act in their best interests and, therefore, happier to accept his treatments. In line with this is Ben-Sira's (1982) finding that the greatest contribution to patient satisfaction was the doctor 'showing devotion'. Thirdly, the doctor-patient relationship may become in itself a valuable source of reinforcement for the patient and compliance is likely to result in the maintenance of contact and warmth to a greater extent than non-compliance. Fourthly, and finally, if the patient perceives the doctor as kindly and well-meaning (s)he is likely to want to reciprocate, and compliance may be seen as a way of doing this; alternatively, non-compliance may be a mark of contempt. With the exception of the last, all these routes can, at a pinch, be subsumed by the HBM.

HEALTH LOCUS OF CONTROL

The possibility that health locus of control orientation (see Chapter 2 for an introduction to this concept) might influence compliance has interested many researchers (see Wallston and Wallston, 1982, for a review). However, as Wallston and Wallston conclude, 'research using the Health Locus of Control (HLC) and Multidimensional Health Locus of Control Scales (MHLC) continues to provide conflicting data'. Some studies report no relationship between health locus of control dimensions and compliance (e.g. Nagy, reported in Wallston and Wallston, 1982) while others variously report a positive association of the powerful others scale of the MHLC and compliance (e.g. Hatz, 1978; Goldstein, 1980), the internal scales of the MHLC and HLC and compliance (e.g. Wallston and McLeod, reported in Wallston and Wallston, 1982; DeVellis et al, 1980b; Goldstein, 1980), and the external scale of the HLC and compliance (e.g. Key, 1975). The chance scale of the MHLC, generally, has not been found to be associated with compliance (see Wallston and Wallston, 1982).

There do not appear to have been any studies looking at simple health locus of control scale scores and compliance in RA. One prospective study (Lorig et al, 1985) which assessed both health locus of control (using the HLC) and the practice of self-management behaviours (as distinct from compliance) did not report the association of these variables, although they did report finding that while self-management behaviours increased, as a result of the educational intervention, locus of control was unchanged.

One possible explanation for the seeming inconsistency of results is concerned with the issue of the dimensionality of health behaviour raised earlier in this review. Certain behaviours, such as adherence to diets, practice of exercise, etc., require a considerable amount of self-control and a belief by the individual in their ability to control their own health (internal orientation) is likely to both affect and reflect adherence. Adherence to behaviours which require less personal control (e.g. medication compliance) are likely to depend more on patients' beliefs in powerful others. The pattern of results, although, by no means very clear, is generally in line with this analysis, and certainly this possibility is worthy of further study.

The Health Locus of Control Typology

The Possibility that the health locus of control typology, proposed by Wallston and Wallston (1982) and described in Chapter 2, may be helpful in understanding compliance and health behaviour in general, remains largely unexplored. A search of the literature revealed no relevant studies and personal communication (1986) with the proponents of the typology brought to light only one unpublished study (Roskram, 1986), which, remarkably, was conducted on a sample of RAs.

Roskram utilized a longitudinal design to examine differences among patients in different categories of the typology (N.B. only categories one to five were examined) in terms of their response (compliance and adjustment) to illness flare-ups. She reports that frequency of flare-ups had the greatest effect on the self-reported compliance of the pure internals (high IHLC, low PHLC and CHLC), who reported less adherence following a high frequency of flare-ups.

PATIENT KNOWLEDGE

Recurrent throughout the topics considered in this chapter is the theme of patient knowledge or beliefs, hence, I propose to close the chapter with a short review of this area.

THE ADEQUACY OF PATIENT KNOWLEDGE

Ley (1982a) distinguishes three criteria most frequently used to assess the adequacy of information given to patients, namely: (1) the extent to which patients are satisfied with the information they are given (2) the extent to which patients know what their physicians wish them to; and (3) whether patients actually have information that the researcher considers they should have. Using any of these three criteria, patient knowledge is woefully inadequate. For example, across the studies Ley considers, dissatisfaction with information or communications ranged from 8-65%, the median level being in the mid-thirties. Dissatisfaction is high across different groups of patient, including: hospital inpatients (Ley et al, 1974, 1976a; Raphael and Peers, 1972; Parkin, 1976), out-patients (e.g. Fisher, 1971) and general practice patients (e.g. Ley et al 1976b); surgical (Ley et al, 1974), medical (Ley et al, 1976a), maternity (e.g. Jolly et al 1971) and psychiatric patients (Raphael and Peers. 1972); and in both the U.S. (e.g. De Castro, 1972) and U.K. (e.g. Ley 1976b). Ley (1982a) also notes that there is no indication that dissatisfaction is abating - more recent surveys indicate no less dissatisfaction than earlier ones.

Evidence that this dissatisfaction is justified is provided by studies which have actually assessed patient knowledge. Svarstad (1974), for example, found that a sizeable proportion of his sample did not know very elementary facts about their regimens, such as how often to take their medications. It is also the case that sizeable proportions (between 14 and 69%) of patients do not even know their diagnosis (Grennan et al, 1978; Ellis et al, 1979; De Castro, 1972). Again, this pathetic picture is common to patients with a variety of illnesses, including the mothers of paediatric patients (De Castro, 1972), general medical patients (Ellis et al, 1979) and arthritics (Grennan et al, 1978). Grennan et al, in fact, reports that 14% of their general arthritic sample (osteoarthritics, rheumatoid arthritics (RAs) and ankylosing spondilitis patients), and indeed 14% of RAs, were unaware of their diagnosis; 36% (31% of RAs) did not know the names of their drugs; just under 75% on non-steroidal anti-inflammatory (NSAI) drugs were unaware of the major side-effects of these drugs; and less than 31% of RAs on the potentially more toxic second-line anti-rheumatic drugs had any idea of the sort of symptoms that might indicate drug toxicity. Most patients, asked if they thought their drugs would cure their arthritis, said 'no'; 9% of RAs on NSAI and 8% on disease modifiers thought they would. Incidentally, this is the only study of RAs in which the content of patient knowledge is actually reported and these are the only results reported.

WHY DO PATIENTS KNOW SO LITTLE?

It seems likely that poor patient knowledge arises for a number of reasons, including:

(1) lack of patient understanding and recall of what they are told;

(2) poor communication techniques of physicians;

(3) patient reticence;

(4) lack of physician commitment to giving information; and

(5) lack of consideration and insensitivity of physicians to patients' needs.

Lack of Patient Understanding and Recall

Various methods have been used to assess patients' understanding and memory for what they have been told or given to read, namely: self report (e.g. Korsch et al, 1971; Kincey et al, 1975; Ley et al, 1975; Ley et al 1976b); clinician judgement (e.g. Ley and Spelman, 1967; De Castro, 1972; Ellis et al, 1979); direct tests (Roter, 1977; Mazzullo et al, 1974; Riley, 1966; Hermann, 1973; Boyd et al, 1974; Parkin et al, 1976); and by the application of readability formula to written information (Ley and Morris, 1984; Ley et al, 1972; Ley, 1974; Liguori, 1978; French et al, 1978; Pyrczak and Roth, 1976). In a review of the research Ley (1979a, 1982a, 1985) concludes that between 35 and 92% of patients do not understand information they are given and between 12 and 69% (median 43%) of information given is forgotten.

Poor Communication Techniques of Physicians

A good proportion of responsibility for patients' lack of understanding and memory for the medical information they are given during consultations must surely lie with the physicians presentation of material. Many medical schools do not systematically teach doctors how to present material to patients, yet it seems likely that adherence to a few simple principles or techniques of information presentation would produce quite rewarding results in terms of increased patient recall and understanding.

A variety of techniques or methods of presentation have been shown to improve recall of orally given information, including: the use of the primacy effect (Ley, 1972); stressing of importance (Ley, 1972); categorization of information (Ley, 1979b; Ley et al, 1973); simplification (Ley, 1982b; Ley et al, 1972; Bradshaw et al, 1975); repetition, both by the information giver and by the receiver of information (Ley, 1979b; Kupst et al, 1975; Bertakis et al, 1975); and by the use of specific, rather than general advice statements (Bradshaw et al, 1975). Improvement in recall has been reported as ranging from 20 to 219% (Ley, 1982a).

Patient recall is also likely to be improved by a number of other methods - which doctors very seldom employ - such as providing patients with written information (see Morris and Halperin, 1979, for a review of the effectiveness of this method) or a tape recording of the consultation (Butt 1977; Reynolds et al, 1979) or relevant audio-visually presented material (Midgley and Macrae, 1971). The points (e.g. simplification, categorization etc.) underlined as being important in the provision of oral information are also likely to be important facets of these alternative methods of information presentation, although there is some evidence to suggest that written information should not be too simplified (Ley et al, 1972).

Patient Reticence

Part of the explanation of why patients remain so ill-informed probably relates to their reticence to ask questions and demand information of their physicians and other health care providers.

Arguably, this reticence on the part of patients stems primarily from the social roles assumed by both the doctor and patient. According to Parsons (1951) the physician is 'an agent of social control' charged by society with the task of returning the ill person to being a fully functioning member of society. As Parsons sees it, in order to perform this function it is necessary for the physician to have power and authority over the patient. This power and authority is achieved by virtue of the professional prestige of the practitioner, the situational authority of the practitioner, and the situational dependency of the patient. The professional prestige of the physician stems from the fact that (s)he has undergone extensive training and is consequently highly skilled and knowledgeable and also from the fact that (s)he is the minister of health, a highly valued 'commodity'. The situational authority of the physician refers to the fact that s(he) enjoys something of a monopoly over health care, while the situational dependency of the patient refers to the fact that the patient needs or is dependent on the care of the physician. Relating to this latter point, according to Parsons' (1951) formulation of the sick role, individuals who accept or assume the sick role, in return for being excused their normal obligations to society - i.e. work and other roles and responsibilities - take on two new obligations, namely: to try and get well and to seek the help of competent helpers (in our society, physicians are the 'ordained healers'). Thus, the institutionalized social roles of doctor and patient tend to lead or bias the patient towards being a relatively passive recipient of care provided by an authoritative physician. Furthermore, there is evidence that physicians commonly discourage patients from asking too many questions (see below).

Patients in the lower socio-economic groups are particularly likely to be diffident in asking for information from their physicians (Waitzkin and Stoeckle, 1972; Pendleton and Bochner, 1980). Bochner (1983) suggests this is because of the 'cultural distance' and 'status imbalance' between doctor and patient, which he suggests leads to 'diffidence and awkwardness' on both sides.

There have been some attempts to counter patient reticence. Roter (1977) gave patients, what amounts to, assertion training. First she ascertained what it was they wished to find out from their doctors and then, utilizing didactic instruction and rehearsal, she taught patients how to ask their doctors for this information . Patients given this intervention did ask more direct questions of their doctors in the following consultation and interestingly, were more likely to attend for follow-up treatment.

Lack of Physician Commitment to Giving Patients Information

On top of patient problems in understanding, remembering and asking for information, and the poor presentation of information, evidence suggests that many doctors are reluctant to give information, or at least, spend very little effort or time doing so. Direct observation of consultations and analysis of consultation transcripts indicates that patients are frequently given very little information. Looking at consultations involving general practice patients, Webb (1976) concludes that all 50 patients in the sample received inadequate information concerning their treatment. Similarly, Stavstad, (1974) reports that in 63% of 221 consultations patients were not given adequate information about their treatment.

Doctors typically suggest a number of reasons why they withhold information from patients. These reasons include a lack of time on their part and the belief that some types of information, such as information about drug side-effects or a poor prognosis, might unnecessarily worry or upset patients or lead to non-compliance. Evidence refutes these reasons. Studies which look at the reactions of terminally ill patients, or patients with cancer, to information about their prognosis indicate that, generally, they approve of being told (e.g. Gilbersen and Wangensteen, 1962; Kelly and Friesen, 1950; Aitken-Swan and Easson, 1959) and Gerle et al (1960) found that terminally ill cancer patients informed of their prognosis actually showed better adjustment. Where information is given about the possible side-effects of treatment the effect has generally not been to increase either reporting of side-effects (Eklund and Wessling, 1976; Paulson et al, 1976; Suveges, 1977; Weibert, 1977) or non-compliance (Myers and Calvert, 1973, 1978). Finally, there is evidence that providing people with good health information actually reduces the total number of visits they make to the physician (Lorig et al, 1985), a finding which suggests providing patients with information may be economic in terms of physician time.

Some (see for example, Nichols, 1983; Waitzkin and Stoeckle, 1972) have suggested other reasons why doctors may deliberately withhold information from patients, reasons concerned with the personal needs and desires of physician to protect their position of power and also to protect themselves legally. Arguably, as the competence gap, or knowledge gap, between practitioner and patient is reduced so is the physician's position of power and prestige. Similarly, the more patients know or understand what is going on, what should be going on, and what alternatives are available in the way of treatment, the more likely they are to recognise the inevitable incidences of professional mismanagement, negligence and incompetence, common knowledge of which will both reduce the omnipotent status of the doctor and leave him/her liable to prosecution. These selfish reasons for restricting the amount of information patients get may not be conscious but rather are incorporated or assumed in medical socialization and training.

Lack of Consideration and Insensitivity of Doctors to Their Patients' Needs

The classic satirical doctor-patient scenario is of the physician writing out a prescription as the patient steps over the threshold into the consulting room, and before even glancing at the patient. The physician behaviour caricatured in this type of scenario has been variously termed 'doctor-centred' (Byrne and Long, 1976) 'doctor-dominated' (Shuy, 1974) and 'bureaucratic, task-oriented' (Plaja and Cohen, 1968). According to researchers in the area, this form or style of doctor-patient interaction is the most common (Plaja and Cohen, 1968). The 'doctor-centred' physician is task oriented, single-minded, dominant, insensitive, inconsiderate, unresponsive, and unrevealing and the antithesis of the 'patient-centred' physician who has been characterized as being 'silent, listening and reflecting' (Byrne and Long, 1976).

There are probably a number of reasons why the 'doctor-centred' style of interaction is so common. First, feigned or ingenuous insensitivity is a convenient way of avoiding giving patients information - reasons physicians might find this desirable have already been considered. Secondly, two aspects of the ethos of the medical profession, proposed by Parsons (1951), are likely to result in insensitivity, namely: 'affective neutrality' and 'functional specificity'. Doctors are supposed to remain objective so that their judgement is not compromised (Leif and Fox, 1963) and also, arguably, do so for their own psychological well-being (Nichols, 1983). They are also supposed to restrict themselves to a consideration of the patients medical or physical condition as this is their area of expertise. The 'doctor-centred' doctor is arguably too objective or detached and too task oriented. The ideal balance of 'detached-concern' (Lief and Fox, 1963) is not easy to achieve in practice. Finally, as mentioned in the preceding section, doctors learn to interact with patients mainly by example and experience, hence, this style of interacting is likely to be self-perpetuating.

CHAPTER 4

UNORTHODOX TREATMENT USE

INTRODUCTION

Compliance with a medical regimen represents just one aspect of 'illness' behaviour. A whole range of other 'illness' behaviours can be subsumed under the general heading of unorthodox treatment (UT) use.

For the purpose of this review UTs may be considered to be treatments not recognized by the orthodox medical community as appropriate for the condition for which they are being used. In Britain this includes treatments such as homeopathy, acupuncture, naturopathy, osteopathy, reflexology, herbalism, Alexander technique, mental imagery and aroma therapy, to mention just a few of the most common and defined types. It also includes more obscure behaviours such as the wearing of copper bracelets and rubbing on of strange 'cocktails', folk remedies and the use of preparatory medicines for conditions other than they were intended, e.g. using laxatives for the treatment of arthritis. A detailed account of some of the most common unorthodox practitioner treatments can be found in Salmon (1984) and the British Medical Association (BMA) report on UTs (1986).

The whole gamut of UTs have been applied and used by RAs (see Kronenfeld and Wasner, 1982). Arthritis has no known cure, yet it is a very painful condition which often leaves people desperate for a cure or at least a palliative. Arthritis in one form or another affects a great many people (approximately 1-2% of the population suffers from RA) and most people experience rheumatic pain at some time or other. Hence, an arthritis treatment has a potentially huge market and there has been no reticence in filling that market need. Unorthodox cures and remedies abound for arthritis and the relevant shelves in book shops and health food shops are well stocked with literature recommending their use.

Another factor which makes RA sufferers a particularly good 'target' is the nature of the disease itself (Consumer Report, 1979). RA is characterized by variability - flare-ups in disease activity followed by periods of remission or relative remission. A period of relief following the initiation of a new treatment may well have nothing to do with the treatment but it is easy to understand how someone desperate to establish control over a very painful condition might be bias to perceive a contingency where none existed. Thus, not only are sufferers very likely to come across literature expounding the virtues of UTs but they are also quite likely to meet people for whom UTs 'really worked'. Arthritis sufferers are also likely to be encouraged to try UTs by friends, family and even slight acquaintances - folk cures for arthritis and rheumatism are so widely known that practically everybody knows of an UT that they will 'swear by' or at least that somebody they know will 'swear by'!

The use of UTs is very widespread and, especially if one considers all the self-care and folk remedies that are used, far exceeds the use of conventional medical treatment (CMT) (Wolinsky,1982). Coe (1978) estimated that over $50 million a year is spent on UTs in the U.S.. Far from it being a minority of eccentrics or only certain ethnic groups or cultures who use UTs it is slowly being recognised that UTs are used by a great many 'normal' westerners (Wolinsky, 1980; Casel, 1976; Riley, 1980). With specific regard to arthritis a study commissioned by the Arthritis Foundation (Walrad, 1960) reported that approximately 50% of arthritics (U.S. sample) questioned used 'unproven' treatments. Kronenfeld and Wasner (1982) suggest this figure is likely to be an underestimation of the true magnitude of use. First, patients were drawn from the mailing list of the Arthritis Foundation and may have been influenced by literature warning against the use of UTs sent to them by the Foundation. Secondly, the data was collected by mailed questionnaire and, hence, presumed a certain degree of literacy, but it has been suggested (although there is little evidence to support it - see below) that UT users are less sophisticated than the users of solely CMTs. Also the response rate was only 31% and, therefore, the sample cannot be assumed to be representative, although the direction of bias likely to result from this can not be anticipated. In their own research Kronenfeld and Wasner found 94% of arthritis sufferers (N=98, 60 RAs) had used an unorthodox remedy or practitioner (80% lotions; 54% diets; 24.5% vitamins; 37.8% jewellery; 12% trips; and 36% an unorthodox practitioner) on average each person having tried 3.7 different remedies (S.D. 2.8).

In terms of the academic literature on UTs, papers are few and far between and hard to locate. A computer search of Psychological Abstracts and

Index Medicus for the period 1967-1985 and 1973-1985 respectively revealed only 11 papers concerned with UTs. These were all obtained from the Medline Database and eight of these papers comprised a series of descriptive reports in the nursing journal Nursing Times. However, 1986 heralded the inclusion of the category 'Alternative Treatments' in Index Medicus - there is no such heading in Psychological Abstracts. Arduous searching for more obscurely categorized papers and the assiduous following of leads (references in obscurely categorized papers) has revealed a very moderate collection of relevant articles.

There have been some papers reporting the dangers of UT use (Rees and Soheed, 1975; Brooks and Lowenthal, 1977; Blackburn and Hindmarsh, 1976; BMA, 1986); others merely describing various types of UT and discussing their underlying philosophies, differences and similarities (e.g. Salmon, 1984; Aasker, 1986; Freer, 1985; Rose-Neill, 1976; Dove, 1976; Snellgrove, 1976; Krieger, 1976; Wilcox, 1976; Edwards, 1975; Harling, 1975; Rigby, 1975); and a few reporting studies of the efficacy of various more common UTs such as acupuncture (see Maddocks, 1985; and Bhatt-Sanders, 1985, for a review), chiropractic (Maddocks, 1985), and homeopathy (Gibson et al, 1980). As to the question of why people should choose to use UTs and the related question, which people use UTs, Butler (1980) reports that a literature search revealed only three relevant empirical papers. I have managed to find a few more papers - mainly post 1980 - even so, it should be said, that the quality and diversity of research and reports is not very good and generally, at least seemingly, unguided by any theoretical considerations.

LIMITATIONS OF RESEARCH ON UNORTHODOX TREATMENT USE

Apart from the comparatively small number of studies, the research conducted so far on UT use is limited in a number of ways.

1. Not many different types of UT have been examined. Only one study (Kronenfeld and Wasner, 1982) considers the more obscure types of UT practised unsupervised by the individual at home; most consider unorthodox practitioner use. By far the most researched type of UT is chiropractic and there are reasons for considering chiropractic atypical of the majority of UTs, or rather of considering chiropractic to be more similar to CMT than most types of UT. First, it is perhaps the UT most accepted

by the medical profession. Some physicians actually recommend chiropractic to their patients and a sizeable proportion of chiropractors are in fact medically qualified (Riley, 1980; BMA, 1986). Furthermore, many of the techniques used by chiropractors are used by conventional medicine professionals (typically physiotherapists). Indeed, Butler (1980) compared chiropractor, nutritional counsellor and CMT users and found chiropractor users more similar to CMT users on a number of variables.

2. Most studies have only considered one type of UT; few compare users of different types of UT (see Cassileth, 1984; Butler, 1980; Counte et al, 1978; and Kronenfeld and Wasner, 1982 for exceptions). Yet there is some limited evidence to suggest that different variables are important in predicting different types of UT use (see later section for this evidence)

3. Many comparative studies are confounded. It is not often ascertained that groups of CMT users do not use UTs as well and vice versa. Subjects are typically allotted to groups on the basis of where their name was obtained from - an unorthodox practitioner or conventional medical practitioner.

4. The range of independent variables investigated by researchers is very limited. The most thoroughly researched set of variables are demographic factors. There is little evidence pertaining to the more theoretically interesting independent variables and that there is is typically coincidental or anecdotal in nature.

5. Very few studies report multivariate analyses (for exceptions see Counte et al, 1978; and Butler, 1980). This is obviously a problem in an area such as this where there are many variables likely to be important in explaining behaviour and many variables are likely to interact or correlate.

6. Most of the research is atheoretical. This limitation is related to point four and largely accounts for it.

WHY DO PEOPLE TURN TO UNORTHODOX TREATMENTS?

Many explanations have been proposed to account for the use of UTs. The stance of the medical profession has typically been rather dismissive, defensive and hostile, and has often involved discrediting UTs and their users (e.g. Ballantine, 1972; Relman, 1979). A frequent, although, often tacit, suggestion, is that UT users are in some way less sophisticated than CMT users, or are cranks. It has also been suggested that the use of UTs serves to legitimize an illness which conventional medicine will not recognize or legitimize - thus, UT users are often considered to be fakes or hypochondriacs. Less denigrating to the users are explanations which point to the nature of the treatments themselves and failures or weaknesses in CMT. Evidence, such as there is, pertaining to explanations for UT use will be reviewed below.

THE SOPHISTICATION HYPOTHESIS

Over the past 100 years scientific principles and methodology have remodelled and reshaped the lives of a good proportion of the world's population - the products of 'progress' certainly dominate western society. Not surprisingly, modern medicine, with its scientific basis, has largely superseded more 'primitive' healing systems in western society. UTs which are unscientific (e.g. Relman, 1979), or at least, comparatively unscientific, are generally considered more primitive and, hence, it is not surprising that UT users are also considered more primitive or, put more euphemistically, less sophisticated.

Pertinent to this issue is research which has looked at the demographic characteristics of UT users (for example, socio-economic status (SES), reflecting schooling and occupation, is quite generally accepted as an indicator of 'sophistication') and also more specific research which has looked at the underlying beliefs about illness and life in general of UT users and their knowledge about modern medicine.

The Demographic Characteristics of Unorthodox treatment Users

By far and away the most frequent independent variables in UT use research are demographic variables. As already mentioned, most UT research is seemingly atheoretical but this relative obsession with demographic variables probably reflects, to some extent at least, the tacit adoption of the sophistication hypothesis. Also, in the absence of any theory to guide the selection of independent variables, demographic characteristics are a fairly obvious consideration.

After reading only a few studies examining the demographic characteristics of UT users one is impressed by the inconsistency of findings. Schmitt (1978), reviewing a number of studies looking (often incidentally) at the demographic characteristics of chiropractor users, concludes,

> '.. both the greatest proportion of users to population and greatest frequency of use (or more consistent use) exists at lower-middle income levels.' (p 59).

She also concludes that chiropractor users are likely to be among the moderately educated, female and in the 'younger age category'. (See Schmitt for a review of the studies leading to these conclusions). However, several studies have failed to find a relationship between chiropractor use and demographic variables, including indications of SES (Yesalis et al, 1980; Cleary, 1982; Breen, 1977; Parker and Tupling, 1976; Counte et al, 1978; Kelner et al, 1980). Only two studies, I have come across, suggested chiropractor users are of higher SES than CMT users (Bender, 1965; Kendall and Wolff, 1949) and in both these studies Schmitt (1978) suggests this finding is the result of inadequate/biased sampling.

A similar pattern of inconsistency is found in studies looking at the relationship of demographic variables and use of other types of UT, and interestingly, when a relationship is supported it tends to be in the opposite direction to that predicted by the sophistication hypothesis.

Pruyn et al (1985) found no relationship beween sex, age , income, or education level and adoption of a diet in breast cancer patients, while in their sample of Hodkin's disease patients, sex did significantly differentiate adopters of the diet from non-adoptors - women were more likely to adopt it. Avina and Schneider (1978) report that the homeopathic clients in their sample were predominantly young, white, well educated and holding white collar jobs. Cooper (1983) looking at laetrile (an unorthodox cancer drug) users found them to be mainly middle-class, living in urban areas, having stable jobs, good social support networks and above average education.

Butler (1980) found nutrition counsellor clients to have higher incomes and to be more likely to be a professional or homemaker than chiropractor clients or CMT clients - chiropractor clients were the least likely to be professionals. Nutrition counsellor patients also tended to be older, in fact age significantly distinguished UT users (nutrition counsellor and chiropractic clients) from CMT users. In the discriminant analysis Butler conducted, income significantly distinguished both nutrition counsellor users from CMT users and chiropractor users from nutrition counsellor users. Nutrition counsellor users having the highest income followed by CMT users and then chiropractic users.

In a study of cancer patients Cassileth et al (1984) looked at the following demographic variables: age, sex, race, religion, education, marital status, current members of household, number of family members who had or had had cancer, political preference, and membership of groups or societies. He found only race and education distinguished CMT users from UT users or from UT and CMT users. UT users tended to be white and better educated. This study is fairly unique in that Cassileth et al looked at six categories of UT (all practitioner or treatment centre base, however). The only demographic factor that distinguished users of different UTs was education - users of mental imagery tended to be better educated.

Other studies which compare users of different types of UT in terms of demographic variables are Kronenfeld and Wasner's (1982) and Counte et al's (1978). Kronenfeld and Wasner found no relationship of age, sex, race, geographic location, duration of illness, functional capacity, occupation, education or income with 'magnitude' of use (what is meant by 'magnitude' of use is not made clear - probably it is the number of different treatments tried) in arthritics but income and education were found to be associated with the pattern of use. High income subjects were less likely to use topical remedies, while the low income and education group were more likely to take trips. Diet use was highest in low education groups and lowest in college educated people - a finding opposite to that of Butler, where the types of illness in the sample was heterogeneous, and Cassileth et al (1984), where the sample consisted of cancer patients.

Counte et al (1978) investigated the use of five different types of UT (chiropractic, acupuncture, 'miracle diets', spinal implants and psychic surgery) in a sample of multiple sclerosis patients. They assessed three different categories of variables: social background; utilization and satisfaction with CMT; and illness experience. They regressed these variables on total use of these five types of UT and separately on acupuncture, 'miracle diet' and chiropractic use. Of the demographic variables investigated (SES, income, education, and age) age was the only one to be significantly related to use and that only in the regression on diet use. It seems younger patients were more likely to use diets.

Medical Knowledge and Unorthodox Treatment Use

Schmitt (1978) talks about an 'Inadequate Socialization Theory' of chiropractor use. Basically, this theory suggests that users of chiropractors are people who are ignorant about modern medicine, who simply '..have not been socialized into the legitimate health care system, and therefore, consider a chiropractor as good or even better than a medical doctor' (Schmitt, 1978; p 59). Schmitt, however, rejects this theory. She reports results from a study (Kuby, 1965) which revealed that chiropractor clients know as much about disease symptoms as non-users and are in fact even more favourably inclined towards CMT specialists and use CMT more than non-users.

Counte et al (1978), however, found that knowledge about multiple sclerosis was inversely related to chiropractor use and UT use in general ('miracle diets'; acupuncture; 'psychic surgery'; and chiropractor use). In separate regressions of the independent variables on acupuncture and diet use, 'knowledge of the facts' was not found to be a significant predictor.

The Subcultural Theory of Unorthodox Treatment Use

It has been suggested that one of the reasons UTs are popular is because they offer explanations of illness and treatments which are easy to understand and intuitively appealing (McCorkle, 1961; Cassileth et al, 1984; Kronenfeld and Wasner, 1982; Coulehan, 1985) and a philosophy or approach to healing which is congruent with users beliefs.

Quite a few studies have looked at the use of UTs in other cultures (see for example, Fabrega and Silver, 1973; Leslie, 1974; Schwartz, 1969), where they are not so unorthodox, and related their use to the system of beliefs held. Schmitt (1978), however, concludes (by intuition it seems) that this 'subcultural theory', as she terms it, cannot account for western use of chiropractors. Others do not seem so convinced.

In a paper looking to explain the high use of chiropractors by people living in the middle western state of Iowa, U.S.A., (14% of the population visit a chiropractor each year), McCorkle (1961) describes the Iowonian culture and how chiropractic satisfies certain needs and fits into the belief system of rural Iowonians. Similarly, Helman (1978) quite successfully interprets the use of certain popular folk remedies, in a British sample, in terms of their 'folk model of illness'. According to this folk model, illnesses are either hot or cold and treatments are similarly hot or cold and used to redress the balance or restore the equilibrium.

Quantitative evidence pertinent to this issue is provided by Avina and Schneider (1978) who found that only 19% of their sample said one of the reasons they sought homeopathic treatment was because it was 'consistent with personal principles and beliefs'. Possibly, however, recognition and verbalization of this reason is likely to underestimate its influence.

In both the McCorkle and the Helman studies described above, the populations concerned, although western, were not a random sample of the national population and, arguably, in the McCorkle study, being rural, represented a relatively unsophisticated section of society. However, the thought and philosophy behind some UTs can be seen to be relatively sophisticated. As Cassileth et al state it,

> 'Both the overall orientation and some of the specific practices associated with (modern) unorthodox therapies are consistent with the popular contemporary focus on physical fitness, proper nutrition and improved mental attitudes.' (p 111)

There is perhaps a shift from the more idiosyncratic, superstitious and cranky remedies - often referred to as 'quack remedies' - towards a more systematic and life style oriented approach. Diets, stress management and exercise routines are increasingly being offered as alternative treatments and rather than being less sophisticated than modern medicine these approaches are in line with current medical beliefs and developments. The germ theory of modern medicine, if not actually superseded, is most definitely undergoing modification, with the importance of life-style and stress (the psyche) in the aetiology of disease increasingly being recognised.

The seemingly inconsistent and confusing results obtained with studies examining the sophistication hypothesis may result from this change in emphasis. Some types of UTs may be used by the less 'sophisticated', whereas others may be used by the most 'sophisticated' and 'trendy'. The types of UT Cassileth et al looked at would, according to the above implied definition, be classed as sophisticated (e.g. diets, mental imagery etc.) and users tended to be better educated than non-users. More direct evidence to support this hypothesis is provided by the Butler (1980) study, also reviewed above. In this study, you will recall, chiropractor users were the lowest income group and least likely to be professionals, followed by the CMT group and then the nutrition counsellor group, who were the highest paid and the most likely to be professionals. Arguably, chiropractic, with its emphasis on the practitioner and its simplistic explanation of illness is old fashioned. This issue of the dimensionality of UT use will be returned to in a later section.

THE LEGITIMISATION AND PSYCHOLOGICAL NEEDS THEORIES

It has been suggested that chiropractors meet mainly psychological needs (Wardwell, 1951; Firman and Goldstein, 1975). Wardwell suggest this explains the labelling he encountered of chiropractor clients as 'psychos', 'hypochondriacs' and 'dupes'. He describes the chiropractor client as a 'marginal patient' - suggesting that their symptoms are not legitimised or recognized by conventional medical practitioners. Evidence supporting this hypothesis is rather circumstantial and seems mainly to consist of the fact that chiropractors are predominantly patronized by clients complaining of musculo-skeletal problems, especially back problems (see Schmitt, 1978, for a discussion of this evidence), a condition which is often considered to be psychosomatic. However, in the context of back pain, the label 'psychosomatic' seems mainly to reflect the fact that a physical explanation for the symptoms cannot be found (given the present state of the art of diagnosis) and also that so called 'psychosomatic patients' often seem psychologically disturbed or distressed. The implication, however, is that the physical symptoms are spurious. Alternatively, it could be argued that the label 'psychosomatic' serves, by discrediting the patient, for whom the doctor is impotent, to preserve the 'omnipotent', all powerful status of the doctor and modern medicine. While the observation that these patients seem to be disturbed can be explained as being a natural reaction to the experience of hopeless (medicine can do nothing) pain.

In any event, not all UT users are 'shunned' by conventional medicine. Many people with indisputable physical illness do use UTs and unorthodox practitioners (e.g. Kronenfeld and Wasner, 1982; Counte et al, 1978; Cassileth et al, 1984) and clearly the 'legitimacy hypothesis' cannot explain their use of UTs very adequately. Along the same lines, however, is the hypothesis that UT users are more psychologically disturbed or distressed than non-users.

Cooper (1983) suggests that the findings that 50% of laetril (an unorthodox cancer drug) users had, at some time, seen a mental health professional, supports this latter hypothesis. However, the lack of any control group in this study and the small sample (N=14) makes interpreting this result somewhat difficult. Pruyn et al (1985) found that cancer patients who felt they had been given insufficient or unclear information were more likely to be adoptors of an unorthodox diet. This relationship held especially for 'stress vulnerable' subjects - subjects high in trait anxiety, or having a low self esteem, or reacting to stress with anger, or any combination of these characteristics. Unfortunately, Pruyn et al do not report the straightforward relationship between trait anxiety and diet adoption. Finally, Parker and Tupling (1976) report that the chiropractor clients in their sample were more psychologically distressed, as measured by the General Health Questionnaire (GHQ), than the general population. However, their Neuroticism scores on the Eysenck Personality Inventory were not significantly different from the general population norm and Parker and Tupling suggest the elevated GHQ scores reflect the fact that these patients were in considerable pain (60% gave a desire for pain relief as the sole reason for attending the chiropractor).

DISSATISFACTION WITH CONVENTIONAL MEDICAL CARE

Evidence relating dissatisfaction with three aspects of CMT to UT use is available: dissatisfaction with interpersonal aspects of the doctor-patient relationship, dissatisfaction with information exchange, and dissatisfaction with the treatment. This evidence will be reviewed here and finally, in this section, evidence concerning the relationship of unorthodox treatment use and compliance with CMT will be examined.

The Patient Practitioner Relationship

Shortcomings in the doctor-patient relationship are addressed in Chapter 3 of this book. Here, suffice it to say that the doctor-patient relationship is commonly a problematical one.

That a poor doctor-patient relationship may lead people to turn to unorthodox practitioners is suggested by Avina and Schneider (1978) who report that 45% of their sample of homeopath clients reported a poor experience with conventional medicinal practitioners; and Cooper (1983), who reports that eight out of a sample of 14 laetril users complained of inadequate emotional support during CMT and claimed that their doctor-patient relationship was a source of stress. Unfortunately, neither of these studies had control groups. However, Cassileth et al (1984), looking at use of a variety of UTs by cancer patients, report that CMT only users had the best relationship with their conventional medical practitioner, followed by CMT and UT users and then UT only users. Of course the hostility of the medical profession towards UTs may account for this finding, assuming they knew their patients were using UTs.

Of chiropractor clients, Parker and Tupling (1976) note, that while they saw the chiropractor and M.D. as being equally competent, most felt the chiropractor had greater 'interpersonal skills'. Butler (1980), however, reports the antithesis of this - she found that UT users tended to have a more negative opinion of the competence of their M.D. but not of his 'personal qualities'. Also, in none of the studies which have actually asked subjects why they sought UT (Cassileth et al, 1982; Parker and Tupling, 1976; Avina and Schneider, 1978) has a poor doctor-patient relationship been cited, or at least this reason has not been reported in the papers. This may reflect the understandable reticence patients have about criticizing their doctors.

Satisfaction with Information

Again dissatisfaction with information exchange in the conventional medical consultation is a common finding (see Chapter 3) and the results of two studies suggest that it may be contributing to UT use.

Thirty-three percent of a sample of homeopath clients mentioned one of the reasons they went to a homeopath was because they were seeking improved health education (Avina and Schneider, 1978). This was the second most common reason stated. Eighty-one percent of the sample had been dissatisfied with one or more aspects of CMT and 20% of the sample said that one aspect they had been dissatisfied with was health care education. However, other studies which have asked subjects why they chose an UT (see above) have not found education needs to be a common reason given, at least not common enough to report. Furthermore, just what is meant by 'health care education' is not explained.

The second study which suggests that poor information from conventional medical practitioners might be associated with UT use is the Pruyn et al study, discussed above. At the risk of being repetitive - Pruyn et al (1985) found that followers of an unorthodox cancer diet were more likely to be dissatisfied with the quality or clarity of information they had been given by conventional medical practitioners than non-followers.

Satisfaction with Conventional Medical Treatments

Patients may be dissatisfied with the treatment itself for a number of reasons. For example, they may feel it is not working or not working sufficiently (in terms of the Health Belief Model (e.g. Becker and Rosenstock, 1984), the value of treatment is low); they may be put off by the side-effects or the risks of side-effects associated with a treatment, or they may feel it costs too much in some other way - for example, in money, time, commitment, discomfort etc..

Both Wolinsky (1982) and Schmitt (1978) have suggested that people are more likely to use UTs when their illness is hopeless or more specifically not amenable to CMT. In line with this is the suggestion that people turn to UTs when they feel their CMT is not working (Koos, 1967; Kuby, 1965; Elder and Acheson, 1970). That this is so is attested to by the fact that unorthodox practitioners are usually consulted for more chronic conditions and usually after CMT has been sought (Butler, 1980; Kronenfeld and Wasner, 1982). More direct evidence is provided by a number of those studies which have asked patients why they turned to UTs.

For 6% of Cassileth et al's UT users the impetus to seek UT was being told by their physician that they were terminally ill. UT users were also considerably more likely to feel that CMT for cancer was 'useless' or 'more harm than good'. Fifty-five percent of Avina and Schneider's (1978) sample claimed the reason, or one of the reasons, they sought homeopathic treatment was their belief that CMT was failing. Similarly, in a study of chiropractor patients, Parker and Tupling (1976) found that 82% of the sample had received and failed to respond significantly to previous treatment (mainly CMT) and two-thirds said they visited the chiropractor as a last resort. Counte et al (1978) found multiple sclerosis patients who were satisfied with the hospital were less likely to use UTs. However, patients were more likely to try chiropractors if they were satisfied with their CMT multiple sclerosis centre. Unfortunately, Counte et al do not indicate what aspects of satisfaction comprised their CMT satisfaction measure. Additionally, they report that disability (arguably, the inverse of treatment success) was a significant predictor of chiropractor use, acupuncture use and overall UT use. It was not a significant predictor, in regression, of diet use however.

With regard to the question of it being the costs of CMT pushing people towards UTs, there is little evidence. Cassileth et al (1984), however, do report that the most popular answer of UT users to the question of what attracted them to UT was that it was 'non-toxic' or 'natural'. Avina and Schneider (1978) also note that 55% of the homeopath clients in their sample reported being dissatisfied with the drug side-effects they had experienced under conventional medical care and 83% of users said the reason they turned to homeopathy was 'seeking relief of a problem without traditional medicine' - whether this was explicitly to avoid the side-effects of CMT is not made clear.

As far as monetary costs go, in Britain, at least, UTs are generally going to be more expensive than CMT, as even across the counter herbal remedies are typically more expensive than a prescription. In other western countries, where medical care is a personal expense, a monetary incentive may be involved in UT use.

Compliance and Unorthodox Treatment Use

Using UT has been considered to be a deviant practice (e.g. Vissing and Petersen, 1981; Aakster, 1986), hence, it is rather surprising that no study has really been addressed to investigating the relationship of unorthodox treatment use and compliance with CMT. Two studies touch on this issue incidentally. Cooper (1983) reports that five out of 15 users of laetril had either refused or discontinued CMT. Similarly, Cassileth et al (1982) note that of patients who used both UTs and CMTs for their cancer, 40% discontinued CMT entirely in favour of UT. Of the 60% who used UT and CMT in conjunction, Cassileth et al do not report whether they were more or less compliant with CMT than CMT only patients. In many of the studies on UT use, whether users are using CMTs as well is not reported. The two studies which actually look at UT use by conventional medical clients (Kronenfeld and Wasner, 1982; Counte et al, 1978), unfortunately, do not address this issue. Clearly, this is an issue in need of more research.

One other study (Butler, 1980) has looked at the relationship of UT use and other health behaviours. Butler reports that UT users are more likely to practice preventive health behaviours than M.D. patients (e.g. to watch their weight). However, this variable was not a significant predictor on discriminant analysis.

THE PULLING POWER OF UNORTHODOX TREATMENTS

So far this review has tended to look at explanations for UT use which are rather negative in connotation. It has been suggested that UT users are less sophisticated and that the problems of modern medicine drive people away, towards an alternative. By way of redressing the balance, some of the positive, pulling aspects of UTs will be considered in this section.

The Treatment

In their favour most UTs are relatively free of side-effect - although the BMA (1986) report on UTs does document a number of risks - and certainly, the naturalness, harmlessness, and wholesomeness of UTs tends to be emphasized in their marketing.

Some UTs are intrinsically pleasant (e.g. some herbal remedies, massage, heat, aroma therapy), although many, the consensus of opinion would surely feel, are not (e.g. acupuncture, manipulation, some herbal remedies).

Related to this last point, many UTs involve physical contact between the practitioner and client and this physical contact has been suggested as being an important component of the therapeutic relationship (Coulehan, 1985) and one which is largely missing in CMT, where , with the exception of physiotherapy, physical contact tends to be largely confined to diagnosis and specifically, to rectal and vaginal examinations, where discomfort and embarrassment (on both parts) are the overwhelming experience. Coulehan (1985), talking about chiropractors, stresses the importance of physical contact, suggesting it gives patients a 'prolonged experience of something happening to the body' (p 388). He also points to the dramatic aspects of chiropractic manipulations, which are often accompanied by a 'click' or 'snap' and which he suggests are 'more immediate and have greater symbolic value to the patient than pills or behavioural instructions'(p 388). In addition to the impact of physical treatment such as chiropractic, touching in itself is likely to help foster a warm relationship.

The Practitioner-Patient Relationship

Typically, the unorthodox practitioner spends a considerably greater amount of time on each consultation than the conventional medical practitioner (Avina and Schneider, 1978; Hewer, 1983). Clearly, some UTs, such as chiropractic, acupuncture and others which involve contact treatments, require this. Additionally, the more holistic philosophy common to the majority of UTs (Aakster, 1986) requires a longer consultation. In CMT, once the disease or syndrome has been identified the treatment can be 'read off'. In most UTs each individual is considered to be unique and consequently, their ailments and treatment are also unique - diseases and syndromes are not generally diagnosed. It is not until the practitioner has a complete picture of the individuals health (physical, psychological and social) that treatment can be recommended. The extra time involved and the intensity of questioning and interest the practitioner pays to small details, undoubtedly, do leave most patients feeling satisfied that the practitioner has got the whole story on which to base treatment. It also enables and fosters the establishment of a relationship where information exchange and, indeed, affective exchange, are possible. The practitioner's interest in what their client has to say is also, undoubtedly flattering and pleasing - most people like to talk about themselves.

It has also been suggested that the unorthodox practitioner-client relationship will probably tend to be more egalitarian than the doctor-patient relationship (e.g. Avina and Schneider, 1978) and for many people this is also desirable. This is likely due to the fact that unorthodox practitioners do not hold such an esteemed position in our society as conventional medical practitioners, that the unorthodox practitioner is actually paid directly by the client, and also to the fact that longer consultations do allow client and practitioner to get to know each other better, and familiarity serves to break down barriers, such as those occasioned by role or status.

Optimism and Control

Evidence considered elsewhere in this review supports the contention that unorthodox practitioners are unlikely to admit that a case is hopeless. Clients are unlikely to be turned away with the 'you'll just have to live with it' or 'I'm sorry there's nothing that can be done' comments that doctors have been known to utter. Cynics might suggest avarice is behind this eternal optimism but, if one examines the philosophy of many of the UTs, another explanation is possible. Undoubtedly, part of the explanation lies in the fact, already mentioned, that unorthodox practitioners do not tend to make diagnoses as such and there are no set treatments. Hence, if a treatment fails there are always more to try. Treatment failures are acceptably explained in terms of the individualistic nature of the patient.

Additionally, many UTs explain illness in terms of 'disequilibrium' (e.g. acupuncture) - the body, as it were, has got out on 'sync' and can no longer maintain the balance necessary for health. When in balance the bodies own rejuvenating and healing power maintain health. Consequently UTs involve trying to restore balance so that the body can heal itself. Given such a conceptualization of health and illness (and it is not so different from modern medicine's understanding of the central role of the immune system in maintaining health) no case is hopeless - it is always possible to work towards the achievement of equilibrium.

Evidence that the illusion of control (in the objective absence of control) is preferable to a belief in no control is available (see Langer, 1983). If nothing else an 'illusion of control' is more comfortable than a belief in no control (see Thompson, 1981) and if one accepts the role of the psyche in determining physical health, a belief in control may actually constitute a degree of control.

Locus of Control

Whether a treatment achieves some control over symptoms may not be the only question of importance concerning control, although, it is probably the most important. Possibly also of importance is the question of locus of control (see Chapter 2 for a review of this concept).

Another plus for UTs, that has been suggested (e.g. Coulehan, 1985), is that they encourage a belief in personal control over one's health, something conventional medicine, with its 'omnipotent medic', is rather apt to quash. Certainly, the underlying philosophy of many UTs, outlined above, is in line with the idea of personal control over health. This emphasis on personal control is also becoming more prominent in contemporary UTs.

> '.. contemporary alternatives, unlike the pills and potions of the past (and indeed, of CMT) are long-term life style oriented options that exist within a broad view of health and personal responsibility.' (Cassileth et al, 1984; p 12)

Many of the practitioner dominated alternatives (e.g. acupuncture, chiropractic) are becoming quite eclectic and advice on life style (especially diet and exercise) is very commonly given, regardless of the unorthodox practitioner consulted.

One study has looked at the relationship of health locus of control (operationalized in terms of the Multidimensional Health Locus of Control scales (Wallston et al, 1978)) and utilization of UTs (Butler, 1980). The combined unorthodox treatment users group (chiropractor and nutrition counsellor users) was distinguished from the CMT users, in discriminant analysis, by a lower belief in the affect of chance on their health. However, when chiropractor use and nutrition counsellor use was analysed separately, chiropractor users were distinguished from both nutrition counsellor and CMT users by their low beliefs in chance, while nutrition counsellor users were distinguished by a low belief in the power of others to control their health, and a high belief in personal control (the internal scale). Both nutrition counsellor and chiropractor clients were more likely to engage in preventive health behaviours than CMT users. This result was significant using analysis of variance but practice of preventive health behaviour was not a significant predictor in the discriminant analysis.

These results are as one might anticipate. Both types of UT users are distinguished by a greater belief in control, or at least, less belief in the role of chance. This belief in control may have led to them seeking UT, or alternatively, may have arisen from their having attended an unorthodox practitioner, or possibly, and perhaps most likely, both influences are in operation. The nutrition counsellor users' high belief in personal control and low belief in powerful others, may also have been anticipated as, although seeking the advice of a practitioner (a powerful other), nutrition counsellor clients are seeking to change their diet, a behaviour requiring personal control.

THE DIMENSIONALITY OF UNORTHODOX TREATMENT USE

To date this review has tended to consider UT use as a unidimensional phenomenon, although the possibility that this is not the case has been suggested (see section on Subcultural Theories of Unorthodox Treatment Use). No study has adequately explored the dimensionality of unorthodox treatment use. In fact, only four studies have looked at more than one type of UT use (Cassileth et al, 1984; Counte et al, 1978; Butler, 1980; and Kronenfeld and Wasner, 1982). Some of the evidence from these studies, suggesting that UT use may not be unidimensional, has already been reviewed, however, for the sake of clarity, and at the risk of repetition, these studies will be briefly reviewed again, with the emphasis being on what they say about the dimensionality of UT use.

Kronenfeld and Wasner (1982) looked at UT use in a group of heterogeneous arthritics (predominantly osteoarthritis sufferers) and distinguished five types of UT used by these patients: topical remedies, jewellery, diets, vitamins and trips. They looked at the pattern of usage as a function of just three variables: income, education and disease category. Income and education did not significantly distinguish users of different types of UT - although, people in the highest income bracket were less likely to use topical remedies, while those with the lowest income or lowest education were most likely to take trips. Furthermore, diet therapies tended to be used most in the least educated group and least in the most educated group - a result in opposition to the proposal regarding sophistication and type of UT used, made in the section of this review entitled, 'Subcultural Theories of UT Use'. Most clearly related to the type of UT used was disease category. Patients with both RA and osteoarthritis or those with only osteoarthritis, were much more likely to use vitamin therapies than patients with other types of rheumatic disease (e.g. RA only, ankylosing spondilitus, gout). This pattern was also true for diet therapies but this result did not reach statistical significance. Finally, jewellery was most popular among patients with either RA or with both RA and osteoarthritis.

Cassileth et al (1984) report that 'no set of demographic characteristics characterized cancer patients on one kind of treatment compared with those on other types ', but goes on to say that patients who used mental imagery were 'somewhat' better educated. As is typical in these studies, the precise method of analysis, and the variables included, is not made clear, but probably this analysis comprised a series of chi squared tests and other bivariate statistics. The UTs distinguished in the study, and thus, probably in these analyses, were: metabolic therapy; diet therapy; megavitamins; mental imagery; spiritual therapy or faith healing; and immune therapy. 'Demographic' variables included the following: age; sex; race; religion; education; marital status; current membership of household; no of family members who had died or been diagnosed with cancer; political preferences; and membership of groups or societies.

Details of the methodology and analysis in the Counte et al study are far from adequate. However, basically, it appears Counte et al assessed three types of independent variables in a group of multiple sclerosis (MS) patients: social background characteristics; utilization and satisfaction with medical care; and illness experience (including disability, self rating of adaptation, knowledge of disease, beliefs about the emotional/interpersonal effects of MS and frequency of hospitalization). Each of the three most popular UTs used (acupuncture, diet and chiropractic) were then regressed with the predictor variables. (The use of regression analysis here is somewhat dubious as users of each type of UT were distinguish from non-users in a simple bipolar fashion.) The best predictors tended to be different for each type of UT. The best inverse predictors of acupuncture use were extent of physical disability and the opportunity to consult with other doctors for non-MS needs. For chiropractor use the best predictors were knowledge of the facts (users tended to have less knowledge about MS) and beliefs about the effects of MS. Five other variables in the chiropractic analysis also had significant beta weights indicating that chiropractor users tended to have been hospitalized more frequently for their MS; have more doctors concerned with treating their MS but are less likely to have a separate doctor for non-MS needs; and are less disabled than non-users. With regard to diet use, Counte et al conclude, older patients who regularly saw several doctors for their MS were less likely to have tried a diet therapy, while patients with a doctor for non-MS needs were more likely to have tried an unorthodox diet. Significant correlations between acupuncture use and use of the other two types of UT were obtained but diet use and chiropractor use were not significantly correlated.

The meaning of these results is somewhat confused by the grouping together of users of other types of UT and non-users of UTs in the regressions on individual UTs. The finding that both chiropractor users and acupuncture users were less likely to have a doctor for their non-MS needs, while diet users were more likely to have this facility may reflect the importance of the quality of the doctor patient relationship in instigating use of an unorthodox practitioner. The fact that chiropractor patients were more likely to have several doctors involved in treating their MS supports this interpretation to some extent. This diversification of care, which Duff and Hollingshead (1968) refer to as 'committee sponsorship', is implicated in the alienation of patients (Hauser, 1981). Unfortunately, Counte et al provide no interpretation for their results, and the lack of methodological detail precludes, to a large extent, the possibility of interpretation on the part of the reader.

In many ways the best study of the 'bunch' is Butler's (1980). Butler looked at clients of three types of practitioner - chiropractor, nutrition counsellor and M.D. - using discriminant analysis. The independent variables - variables encompassed under the headings: health background, general background, health attitudes, current health needs, and service evaluation - were entered into the discriminant analysis only if they significantly distinguished the groups using oneway analyses of variance. Large values on the first function identified by the three group discriminant analysis best characterized the clients of nutrition counsellors; who, according to the analysis, tended to be people with a long-standing health need; who had seen more than the average number of health practitioners (unorthodox practitioners and conventional medical practitioners) in the past year; had a low belief in the ability of powerful others to control their health and a high internal health locus of control; had the resources for obtaining health care; and a more negative attitude towards the cost, convenience and professional competence of their M.D.. The second function, which characterized the chiropractor client, described people who also had a long standing health need, greater utilization of health services and a more negative attitude towards the competence of their M.D., but with a low belief in the role of chance or luck in the maintenance of their health, combined with a low internal locus of control score, and being younger and less likely to have resources (lower income) than average.

This study is interesting because it suggests the psychological concept of locus of control may underlie type of unorthodox treatment use. Unfortunately, Butler only looked at two types of UT and the groups are probably quite confounded - most UT users had also used conventional medicine for their current problem and the possibility that users of one type of UT also had used, or even were concurrently using, the other type of UT was not excluded.

CHAPTER 5

PILOT STUDY 1 - AN EXPLORATION OF PSYCHOLOGICAL ISSUES IN RHEUMATOID ARTHRITIS

The psychological literature on physical illness is vast and quite diverse. The study described in this Chapter was conducted in an attempt to focus my attention on areas of relevance for the subject sample, namely, out-patients with chronic RA.

METHOD

In order to fulfil the aim of the study it was necessary to employ a very unstructured interview schedule.

A number of topics were discussed with patients:

(1) their emotional reactions to their illness both now and in the past;

(2) the effect of having RA on their life (e.g. occupation, family role, self care, leisure etc.);

(3) their experience of pain - the Melzack Pain Questionnaire (MPQ; McGill, 1975) was used to help patients describe their pain (the psychometric properties of this instrument are considered in Chapter 7);

(4) the role of stress in the aetiology and progression of the disease;

(5) the reactions of their families to their illness; and

(6) their feelings about their treatment and doctors.

In order to elicit conversation and self disclosure a historical perspective was adopted - patients were asked to remember back to the year before they developed RA and recount feelings then and at other key times.

SUBJECTS

Three male and 15 female patients were interviewed. The mean age of the sample was 46.28 years and the mean duration of illness 13.5 years (range 1.5-35 years). Patients were selected at random from a pool comprised of all RA patients attending the Rheumatology Out-patients' Clinic at the Princess Elizabeth Orthopaedic Hospital (P.E.O.H.) in Exeter.

All interviews were conducted in the patients' own homes and recorded on audio tape. On average interviews lasted one and a half hours.

RESULTS AND DISCUSSION

All the tapes were transcribed and the transcripts examined for recurrent themes. The major findings of this study are outlined below. As the aim of the study was to obtain qualitative, impressionistic data, the presentation of quantitative data in this report will be minimal.

EMOTIONAL REACTIONS TO ILLNESS

Depression

Several patients reported fairly violent emotional reactions in the initial stage of their illness, with feelings of despair and anger dominating and overriding their lives for well over a year. Many others reported fleeting periods of depression, lasting perhaps for only a few hours and occurring with greater frequency in the early days.

At interview most patients seemed reasonably cheerful and adjusted, although, one man was receiving treatment for depression and another patient appeared quite markedly depressed. Additionally, there was a fairly pervasive feeling of hopelessness about their arthritis.

Many patients seemed to express an awareness of the importance of not allowing themselves to get depressed; as one patient put it, '.. you can't let it get you down, although, of course it does a bit sometimes'. The feeling generally was that it would be easy to give into it and get depressed, but that RA was really quite enough to contend with without an overlaying depression.

Frustration and Anger

As one patient said, 'frustration is nine-tenths of RA'. Every patient interviewed talked about the frustrations of RA, and several patients actually admitted to having 'tantrums' at times. It was the 'little things' that were described as being frustrating, things such as being unable to turn taps on, or open a jar of coffee or a tin. Also described as frustrating was the fact that it took much longer to do simple jobs, such as make beds and cook, and for many things having to rely on 'willing but often busy and forgetful' spouses. Anger and resentment, evident in a substantial proportion of the sample, on the other hand, was more associated with major restrictions (i.e. the effects of RA on work and leisure activities).

Guilt

Feelings of guilt were fairly prevalent. Many patients felt they were often too sharp or quick tempered with their families as a result of the pain they experienced or the inherent frustrations of RA. Others felt they held their families back; for example, in terms of the type of holidays they had. Other sources of guilt stemmed from:

(1) their spouses having to take over many of their duties on top of their own;

(2) their changed relationship with their children (many mothers regretted they had not been able to be more physical with their children - often though they felt this loss more for themselves than their children);

(3) not doing as much housework as 'they should' - a strong puritan ethic was evident in many patients;

(4) not being able to work and contribute to the family income;

(5) being miserable and 'moaning all the time'.

Edge on Life

Many patients felt that the RA or the drugs had taken their sharpness, clearness of thought, and motivation. They described feeling more 'muzzy' and less able to cope with life.

Anxiety and Fears

Many patients professed to being the 'worrying type'. A number of specific fears relating to their condition were also evident:

(1) the fear that they would become dependent or very badly disabled;

(2) the fear that they would become disfigured and unattractive, or were already unattractive;

(3) the fear that RA is a genetic disease and that their children may get it;

(4) the fear that people will think they are miserable and 'grumpy' - some patients said that when asked, even by doctors, they would say they were alright regardless of how they felt;

(5) the fear that the drugs they were taking may do 'more harm than good';

(6) the fear that the drugs may stop working and that there would be no alternatives;

(7) the fear that they would have to give up work; and

(8) the fear that a flare-up would never end.

EFFECTS ON LIFE

Most patients had problems with some aspect of everyday life (e.g. dressing, bathing, cooking, housework, etc.) and most reported that having RA had restricted their leisure activities and social life to some extent. With regard to the latter issue, a particular problem seemed to be in planning ahead; the inherent variability of RA means that often plans, made by patients when feeling well, have later to be cancelled because of a flare-up.

A few patients had retired early or given up work as a result of their arthritis. In two instances patients reported being discriminated against, when seeking employment, because of their condition. The effects of reduced employment were reported as being both psychological and financial.

Having RA also affected patients' role in the family.

PAIN

Patients were asked to choose, from among those adjectives listed in the MPQ, those which they felt described their pain. The percentage of patients choosing a word from each class and subclass of adjectives is shown in Table 5.1.

Table 5.1

Percentage of Patients choosing a word from each subclass of the MPQ.

ADJECTIVE CLASS	SUBCLASS NO.	SUBCLASS NAME	% (N=17)
	1	temporal	76.5
	2	spatial	82.3
	3	punctate pressure	76.5
	4	incisive pressure	58.8
SENSORY	5	constrictive pressure	82.3
	6	traction pressure	41.2
	7	thermal	8.2
	8	brightness	47.1
	9	dullness	100
	10	sensory misc.	76.5
	11	tension	82.3
	12	autonomic	41.2
AFFECTIVE	13	fear	52.9
	14	punishment	82.3
	15	affective misc.	58.8
EVALUATIVE	16		94.1
	17		70.6
MISC.	18		70.6
	19		11.8
	20		100

Two main types of pain were distinguished: active and mechanical pain. Active pain is characterized in terms of the following adjectives: hot, burning, tender, sharp, throbbing, aching, gnawing, and penetrating. Mechanical pain depicts the type of pain experienced as a result of the damage already done to the joint, rather than the inflammatory process. This type of pain typically occurs on movement and is a 'sharp', 'wrenching' type of pain, described by one person as similar to the pain experienced in a sprained, but otherwise healthy, joint.

Most patients said they were never completely free of pain or discomfort. At its worst many patients rated the pain as 'unbearable', although some were reluctant to do this , saying, '.. but you always do bear it, what else can you do'. At the time of interview most patients described their pain intensity as 'mild' or 'discomforting'. This intensity seemed to reflect a mixture of mild active pain and mechanical pain and was most frequently described as 'dull', 'aching', and 'nagging'.

Many patients were reticent in their use of the affective pain adjectives. It may be that they did not consider these words 'respectable', alternatively, this may reflect the sentiment, expressed by many about the pain intensity, that 'you learn to live with it'. The affective words that were chosen suggest that the pain of RA is a more 'punishing', 'tiring' and 'gruelling' pain than a very 'frightening' or 'blinding' pain. However, some did describe the very active pain as 'killing', 'vicious' and 'frightful'. Intense pain was reported as being associated with feelings of sadness, depression and despair, the less intense background pain was described as 'wearing' and 'annoying'.

ROLE AND EFFECTS OF STRESS

In over half the sample a major life event or stress was reported as occurring in the year preceding the onset of their RA. However, not all patients saw this event as significant. The stresses included: the birth of a baby; miscarriage; separation from spouse and total change of lifestyle; unhappy reorganization of job; bad relationship with father; 'O' levels; moving away from family and friends; and son's illness and diagnosis of diabetes. In only the latter case, however, did the patient categorically feel this stress had caused her RA, although, interestingly, the spouses of two other patients felt very sure that stress was important in the aetiology of their partner's illness (spouses were present in only four cases).

Several patients felt that stress definitely affected their RA and could cite incidences to illustrate this claim. Again a couple of spouses interjected that they felt stress was important even though their partners were not sure. Only two patients indicated they actually tried to moderate the level of stress in their lives in order to influence their RA. Many others felt stress may be important, but could not be certain and certainly the issue was not particularly salient for these people. Several patients thought that at times of general stress their RA was more of a burden, and one patient actually thought their RA felt better at times of stress, due to the distraction element.

REACTIONS OF FAMILIES

Some patients reported that their arthritis had brought them closer as a family, some that it had made no difference, and some felt it had had a negative effect on their family life. For this latter group the changes necessitated in their family role had led to tension and disagreement. The reactions of children tended to reflect that of spouses.

Several patients reported that their husband's reactions to their illness helped them 'keep things in perspective'. The most important thing communicated in this type of reaction was that the patient was still as highly valued with RA as before. There seemed to be two main ways this information was communicated. One approach was to make light and joke about the problems of RA - for example, one patient told how her husband made her laugh by imitating her 'waddle'. The other approach involved serious discussion and counselling.

Other patients were not so lucky in their spouse's reactions. One patient reported that her husband could not accept the fact that she wore 'ugly shoes' and walked with difficulty, 'like an old woman'. In another case the problem seemed to stem from the fact that the spouse also suffered from a serious illness (kidney failure) which took precedence. Finally, the comments of another spouse, present at the interview, suggested some underlying resentment of the fact that her husband's disability had limited her social and leisure activities. Many patients intimated that at times their families were thoughtless and lacking in understanding.

THE DOCTOR-PATIENT RELATIONSHIP

As a group these patients did not seem overly satisfied with their doctors, either G.P. or consultant, although, not all patients had problems with both and some had problems with neither. Most of the problems were of a predictable nature: lack of proper explanations, doctors not liking questions, patients expected to be too passive. Some patients seemed to feel their doctors were a little cold, unconcerned, insensitive and unfeeling. Often they seemed to feel their doctors did not have much time or sympathy for them and at times felt their doctors found them irritating. Often patients who voiced these complaints countered them with comments such as, '.. but what can they do ..', '.. but they haven't really got the time ..', '.. it's partly my fault, I don't like to bother them with my questions, or take their time'. Thus, it seemed patients did not feel easy making these complaints because they were not sure they had any right to expect more from their doctors, because some of the dissatisfaction they felt was more to do with the uncontrollable nature of the disease than their doctors lack of concern, and probably because they saw the interviewer as a representative of their consultant (needless to say, anonymity was assured). However, two patients did most definitely feel neglected and betrayed by medicine. Both felt not everything was being done that could be done, and that doctors had lost interest in their case because it was 'too late'. Both these patients, understandably perhaps given these percepts, seemed a little bitter towards the medical profession. Additionally, many patients did not seem to feel their G.P. was specialized enough to help with their RA.

The most striking impression communicated, and one that was voiced, in so many words, by one patient, was that the doctors took away patients' hope and instilled feelings of helplessness. Several patients reported incidents where they had come home and cried after a visit to the doctor's. A comment that was particularly implicated in conveying this feeling of hopelessness was, 'you'll have to learn to live with it'. Other researchers have commented on the deflating power of this phrase (Roger et al, 1982). Additionally, many patients reported being discouraged by their doctors in their attempts at self-help. There was a considerable amount of interest in unorthodox treatment (especially diets) but several patients reported that their doctors had been very scathing and dismissive about their use. Another patient said she would like to try unorthodox treatments but felt this would jeopardize her relationship with her doctor. Many patients said they did not tell their doctors about the unorthodox treatments they tried. It was not just on the topic of unorthodox treatments that doctors were dismissive, however, one young woman reported being 'put in her place' when she asked about the development of a new hip joint about which she had read in a newspaper.

Advice to 'slow down' was also reported as contributing to feelings of hopelessness. Having sat in on a number of consultations (in a couple of instances, with patients in this sample) I am able to verify the frequency with which this advice is given. Additionally, it seemed to be presented in a rather negative way; the emphasis being on the penalties of not heeding this advice rather than on the benefits. Furthermore, the unpalatability of this advice was not diluted by information regarding when and how joints could be safely, and indeed therapeutically, used. Overall, it seems RA is presented to the patient as a very negative, or as one patient described it, 'no-no' ('don't do that', 'give up this'), disease.

KNOWLEDGE AND MISCONCEPTIONS

A particularly interesting impression gained in discussion of patients' fears and treatment was that a lack of information and consequent misconceptions about the disease seemed to be contributing to psychological distress, and also, possibly, non-compliance and use of unorthodox treatments. There seemed to be a tendency for patients to overestimate some of the risks of RA, such as: the risk of becoming very badly disabled and dependent; the risk of becoming badly deformed; the chances of the disease developing in offspring; and side-effects of drugs. There also seemed to be a tendency for patients to underestimate the efficacy of treatment. The tendency for the consultant to present advice about exercise in a rather negative way has already been commented on. Additionally, several patients thought their drugs were only palliatives when, in fact, they were taking disease modifying drugs. Similarly, quite a few patients were of the opinion that wrist splints served only a palliative function. In one instance a patient stopped taking a disease modifier, because he felt it was not helping, after taking them for just one month. Not only was he unaware of the function of the drug, but, clearly, also of the fact that it generally takes several months for the particular drug in question to have any effect, and about six months before it produces maximal effect.

Anxiety was also engendered by the fact that patients were uncertain of what symptoms they could expect with their arthritis and what the side-effects of the drugs they were on were. For example, one patient was worried that his depression, which had necessitated his absence from work for several months, was a side-effect of the drugs he was on. He felt himself to be in something of a 'catch 22' situation - the depression was severely debilitating but dropping the tablets might precipitate a relapse in his arthritis which would also be debilitating. Despite mentioning this worry to his doctor, this patient had not been reassured that depression was not a recognised side-effect of the tablets he was on. Another patient was concerned that his symptoms may have been due to cancer rather than RA. He was worried that his condition had either been misdiagnosed or that his arthritis was 'blinding' the doctors to the possibility of his also having cancer. Understandably given this fear, the appearance of a rheumatoid nodule (a lump under the skin), which he was unaware was a symptom of RA, considerably alarmed him. A common disease related symptom that several patients were concerned might be a drug side-effect was tiredness.

Reasons why, in the absence of correcting information, patients might be expected to show this negative bias in their beliefs about their illness and treatment have already been discussed in Chapter 2 of this book.

CHAPTER 6

PATIENTS' KNOWLEDGE AND MISCONCEPTIONS ABOUT THEIR ILLNESS

This chapter describes two studies concerned with establishing what RA patients understand about their illness and what misconceptions about it they hold.

In the first study (pilot study 2) the illness knowledge and misconceptions of a small group of RAs was assessed using an interview schedule comprised of open-ended questions. In the second study knowledge and misconceptions were assessed in a larger sample using a postal multiple-choice questionnaire.

PILOT STUDY 2

In particular to elicit patients' misconceptions about their illness, an interview schedule was developed, containing open-ended questions about RA.

It was noted in pilot study 1, that patients seemed to be overestimating the risks of having RA and underestimating the efficacy of treatments, consequently, several items were developed to allow assessment of this tendency. Specifically, these were questions concerned with prognosis and the function, availability and side-effects of treatments and exercise. One or two other items were added because it was felt patients' beliefs about these issues might also affect them psychologically (e.g. items about the cause of RA and demographic characteristics of sufferers). Other items were included to assess practical knowledge about exercise and the use of splints (again these were topics patients, interviewed in pilot study 1, seemed ill-informed about), and general knowledge about RA, including knowledge about the disease process itself. The major categories and subcategories of questions asked are shown in Table 6.1. It should be noted, however, that categories are not exclusive, some items fall between categories.

Table 6.1

Categories and subcategories of knowledge patients were assessed on.

1. Treatment - Costs and Benefits
   a. Types of treatment (including self-help) available for RA
   b. Function of different types of treatment (drugs, surgery, physiotherapy, occupational therapy, exercise, rest)
   c. Type and likelihood of side-effects of different types of drug treatment

2. Treatment - Practical Aspects
   a. Indication for use of splints, exercise and rest
   b. Regimen instructions or details
   c. Knowledge of joint protection techniques

3. Prognosis
   a. Duration of illness
   b. Likely prognosis with regard to disability, disease activity and deformity
   c. Cues to prognosis

4. The Disease Process and General Knowledge about RA
   a. Body systems affected by RA
   b. Effect of RA on different body systems
   c. Clinical symptoms of RA
   d. Pathology underlying symptoms (pain, stiffness inflammation/swelling, general malaise, deformities)
   e. Aetiology
   f. Characteristics of sufferers (age at onset, sex ratio)
   g. Distinction of RA and osteoarthritis

SUBJECTS

Ss were randomly selected from a pool comprised of all those RA patients attending the out-patients rheumatology clinic at the P.E.O.H. Exeter. In all, 17 patients were interviewed, four men and 13 women. The range in age was from 27 to 68 years (mean, 50). Patients had had RA for between one and 33 years (mean, 9.62 years). The population ratio of women to men sufferers is about 2:1 or 3:1, hence, the proportion of women to men interviewed is representative.

RESULTS AND DISCUSSION

(1) **The Disease Process and General Knowledge about RA**

Question - What parts of the body does RA affect?

As already discussed in Chapter 1 of this book, RA can affect many extra-articular organs and body system. The patients in this sample were clearly underestimating the diversity of pathology. Seven patients believed that RA only affects the joints and two others felt that only the joints and related structures (bones and muscles) were involved. The mean number of body parts mentioned (including the joints) was 2.2 (range 1-4). Other than the joints the most popular answers were the eyes (N=3), heart (N=3), muscles (N=3), bones (N=2) and blood (N=3). Other suggestions were the skin, immune system, chest and menstrual cycle.

Question - Can you tell me anything about the structure of the joints? What they look like inside?

Patients were shown a diagram of a joint and asked to label eight structures. The highest number of structures named was six (N=3), the mean was 3.82. Often patients were able to name structures but could not identify them on the diagram (see Table 6.2). Notably, only two patients mentioned the synovial membrane, the seat of pathology in RA.

Table 6.2

Number of Patients Identifying and Correctly Labelling the Eight Joint Structures

Name of structure	No. naming structure (N=11)	No. correctly labelling structure
Bone	11	10
Cartilage	9	6
Muscle	8	4
Tendon	6	5
Fluid	5	2
Synovial membrane	2	1
Capsule	1	0
Bursa	0	0

Question - How does RA affect the joints?

Answers to this question are summarized in Table 6.3.

Table 6.3

Patients' explanations of the disease process

Disease Process	No. suggesting process
Wearing away of bones	11
Loss of joint fluid	10
Cartilage attacked	8
Idea of precipitation/crystals	6
Inflammation	5
Chemical destruction	4
Too much fluid	3
Other	8

Two major categories of misconception were identified in this analysis. First, six patients suggested that some form of precipitation or crystallization was occurring in the joint, a process which does not occur in RA but is characteristic of gout (another form of arthritis). Secondly, the idea that the joint fluid is decreased or, as it was variously put, 'lost', 'dried up', 'worn away'; in fact, it is generally increased. In some instances the fluid was seen as drying up leaving crystals, which, being sharp, lacerate and wear the joint away, and in others the lack of lubrication was seen as leading to frictional 'wear and tear'.

Question - What causes this symptom?

Pain The major causes of pain expounded are shown in Table 6.4. The correct answers are bone rubbing together and inflammation. Interestingly, of the four patients who suggested inflammation, only two had previously mentioned it with regard to the question of the disease process.

Table 6.4

Patients' explanations of the cause of pain in RA

Cause of pain	No. suggesting this cause
Bones rubbing/wearing	6
Inflammation	4
Lack of lubrication/fluid	3
Don't Know	3
Other	5

Stiffness Explaining stiffness caused more of a problem, possibly because the actual cause (an accrual of fluid in the joint) was not compatible with many patients' understanding of the disease process. Four patients simply did not know the cause of stiffness, while a further six could only give an external cause, that of 'keeping still too long', or from one patient, 'the cold'. Two patients suggested that the joint became 'locked', implying some sort of mechanical entrapment. Interestingly, few patients reverted to the joint fluid for their explanations. Two did, however, one simply stating that the 'joint drying out' caused stiffness and the other, rather appealingly, that the fluid 'sets like jelly'.

Swelling Patients' answers to this question are summarized in Table 6.5.

Table 6.5

Patients' explanations of the cause of swelling in RA

Cause of swelling	No. suggesting this cause
Don't know	7
Exercise	5
- overdoing it	4
- not enough	1
Build-up of:	6
- fluid*	4
- crystals	1
- unknown	1

* correct answer

Tiredness/General Malaise Several patients stated that they were not aware that tiredness was in fact a symptom of RA. Another nine patients did not know the cause of the general malaise and tiredness, leaving only five patients who gave answers. Nearly all the answers given were fundamentally correct and included the ideas that the malaise results from the body 'fighting the disease'; from coping with the pain and disability in everyday life; from the inflammation; and because the disease causes anaemia and affects other body systems.

Deformity Nearly half the patients (seven) did not know what causes deformity in RA. Three were aware that some deformity was the result of destruction of the structure of the joint, although only one mentioned that the structure was bone, and an additional four seemed to be aware that supporting structures such as the tendons and joint capsule were stretched or 'slackened'. Other patients talked about the joints being 'pushed out of shape' because of the swelling and 'coming out of their sockets'.

One patient suggested the deformities were the result of 'muscles hardening into lumps'. This idea of there being some permanent thickening of structure was also proposed by another patient and may be the result of confusing RA with osteoarthritis, in which bony 'spurs' grow on the lateral aspects of the bones and produce characteristic nobbles and bumps.

Question - What is the difference between RA and osteoarthritis? Answers are summarized in Table 6.6.

Table 6.6

Suggested differences between RA and osteoarthritis (OA)

Suggested difference	No. suggesting this difference
Severity	3
- RA worse	2
- OA worse	1
Affects different structures	7
OA caused by wear and tear	2
Exercise important in OA	2
Don't know	1

Question - What do you know about the Rheumatoid Factor?
Rheumatoid factor - autoantibodies which attack the immunoglobulin G molecules - is present in the majority of people with RA and is consequently used in diagnosis. Very high levels of rheumatoid factor tend to suggest the arthritis will be severe, or at least that a severe flare-up is underway or imminent. Most patients in this sample, if not all, would have been tested for it.

In the event, only two patients had heard of rheumatoid factor. Both were aware it could be detected in the blood and one patient suggested further that, although associated with getting the disease, it was not involved in the disease process. This is consistent with current knowledge, as the rheumatoid factor has not yet an identified role in the disease process. Neither patient knew anything else about the rheumatoid factor.

Question - At what age are people most likely to start RA?
The most frequent answers were that it affects people at any age (N=6) or that it tends to affect older people (N=6). Four patients thought it occurred most frequently in the middle years and one patient, early to

middle life (20-40 years).

Question - Are the sexes equally affected?

The majority of patients were correct in thinking that RA is more common in women and their estimates of the ratio of women to men suffers (between 2:1 and 5:1) were pretty accurate. Five patients thought that the sexes were equally affected and only one, a man, that more men than women had RA. Two patients would not commit themselves.

Question - What is the cause of RA?

The main causes that patients suggested are shown in Table 6.7. Most patients suggested more than one cause (mean, 2.35). Notably, over half the sample felt that the way they had used their joints in the past and the type of work they had done was, in part at least, responsible for their arthritis - this is contrary to medical opinion.

Table 6.7

Patients' suggestions about the aetiology of their arthritis.

Suggested Cause	No. of patients suggesting this cause
Hereditary	9
Over use/trauma	6
Cause is not known	6
Damp	5
Stress	4
Virus	3
Other illness	2
Diet	2
Other	3

(2) **Knowledge about Treatments**

Question - What types of treatment are available for RA?

Following this very open-ended question - which typically produced the names of a couple of drugs - patients were asked more specifically about four main types of treatment.

Drugs The number of patients identifying each of the four main types of drug used in RA is shown in Table 6.8. The mean number of drug types identified was 2.06; no one patient distinguished all four types. Eight patients mentioned both disease modifiers and NSAI drugs, the key drugs.

Table 6.8

Number of patients identifying the four key types of drug used in the treatment of RA.

Type of drug	No. identifying this drug
Disease modifiers	12
NSAIs	11
Steroids	6
Analgesics	7

Of particular interest was the question of whether patients were underestimating the value of treatment and this issue is addressed in Table 6.9. Notably, no patient thought the drugs they were on would cure their arthritis.

Table 6.9

What patients thought their drugs did.

	Function ascribed to drug			
Type of drug	Disease modifier	NSAI	Analgesic	Don't know
Disease modifier	6	1	1	2
Steroid	1	1	0	0
NSAI	1	9	3	0
Analgesic	0	0	2	0

Drug Side-Effects Most patients on NSAI drugs knew that gastric problems were a side-effect of this type of medication, although, two patients thought there were no side-effects with this type of drug. Similarly, most patients using them knew of one or two side-effects associated with disease modifiers - typically the undesired effects on the blood and kidneys. The few patients on drugs willing to estimate the frequency of side-effects tended to underestimate the risks. The general lack of knowledge about drug side-effects is notable given the fact that the disease modifier drugs used in RA are among the most toxic in current use in medicine.

Surgery All patients thought surgery was a relevant treatment for RA. Fourteen mentioned joint replacement surgery and all but one of these was aware that not all joints could be replaced. Other types of surgery mentioned were: the correction of deformities; tendon repair; insertion of plates in the knee; removal of bunions and toes; and arthrodesis - procedures with which patients had personal experience.

Splints With the exception of one patient everyone had got a least one type of splint - 15 night splints and 13 day splints. Patients with splints were asked what they thought their intended function was (see Table 6.10) and when they thought they should be worn.

Table 6.10

Patients' beliefs about the intended function of their splints.

	Ascribed function				
Type of splint	Reverse deformity	Prevent deformity	Aid perf-mance	Reduce pain	Other
Day	1	6	4	2	3
Night	0	11	1	6	3

With regards the question of when splints should be used, for day splints the most popular answer was, the correct one, that they should be used for work, especially heavy manual work. Some patients felt they should be worn all the time, and one thought they should be used after she had done a lot of work! Most patients felt that night splints should be worn every night. Only a few patients noted that splints were particularly important when the joints were bad.

Rest and Exercise With the exception of one patient who thought no exercise was good and one who thought rest was bad, all patients seemed to have fundamentally the right ideas about exercise and rest. Rather vague statements such as, 'do things in moderation, 'don't over do it', 'gentle exercise', 'if it hurts don't do it' and 'it's important to keep active', were very prevalent, but more specific knowledge about exercise and rest was in most cases difficult to extract, despite the fact that 11 patients had seen a physiotherapist for their RA.

Five patients were unsure about the type of exercise they should be doing and never did any special exercises for their arthritis - surprisingly, only one of these had not seen a physiotherapist. Exercise(s) that are generally beneficial (e.g range of motion, strengthening, swimming) were described by 10 patients. However, two of these patients, along with one other, also mentioned exercise which can be damaging (e.g knitting, sewing and walking).

Ideally it is thought an inflamed joint should be moved through its full range of motion twice daily in order to maintain function but otherwise rested in order to prevent long-term joint damage and the exacerbation of inflammation. Most patients admitted to feeling uncertain about exercising a particularly active joint and, although all but one patient realised it was important to rest it more than usual, only one got the balance of rest and exercise correct (using the above criteria), the rest were equally split between those who recommended absolute rest and those who recommended too much exercise.

Three patients could not suggest a function for either rest or exercise. The majority (13) were aware that the function of exercise is to keep the joint mobile. One of these patients also thought that if they did not exercise when their arthritis was bad the disease activity would be prolonged (an unlikely relationship). The most popular function assigned to rest was that it actually helps ease disease activity. Six patients expressed this in a straightforward way, while two others said that 'overdoing it' produced a flare-up, which is perhaps not quite the same thing. Other answers were that rest enables 'the tissues to recover from overactivity' and that unless one rested during a flare-up the 'white structures' (tendons, joint capsule etc.) would be damaged and consequently deformity produced. One other patient, when asked about preventing deformity, also mentioned the value of rest. All of these ideas are in line with medical opinion and suggest that rest serves more than just a palliative function. However, four patients did think that rest was only a palliative and one was unsure how it helped or even if it helped.

Question - Can deformities be prevented or reversed?
In total 13 patients thought that splints helped to prevent deformity, although only seven mentioned splints when asked this specific question. Exercise and drugs were the next most frequently suggested methods for preventing deformity and rest was also mentioned by a couple of people. Other answers include: diet, warmth, care in lifting things, keeping weight down, surgery and nothing.

Of the 11 asked, five thought that deformities could not be reversed while another five thought that they could via injections (N=2) and surgery (N=3). One thought that deformities would reverse naturally when the disease activity lessened. In fact, for the most part, deformities cannot be reversed.

(3) **Prognosis**

Question - How, if at all, does the disease activity change over time?
The 16 patients asked this question were equally split between four answers: activity stays about the same over time, activity gets worse, activity gets less, and 'don't know'.

Question - Can the activity of the disease ever stop?
Three patients thought that in RA the disease activity never stops. Eight thought that it could sometimes stop but if it was going to stop and when, was unpredictable; two thought that it sometimes stopped after many years and one thought if it was going to stop it would do so early on. Finally, three patients felt that the disease activity did stop but only when the joint was completely 'shot'.

Question - Can prognosis be predicted and if so how?
Six patients thought prognosis could not be predicted and two were unsure one way or the other. Four patients thought prognosis could be predicted, to some extent, by a blood test and three reckoned that if the arthritis

was particularly virulent at first this was a bad omen - in fact it tends to reflect a good prognosis. Symptoms first presenting in the hands one patient thought was an indication that the arthritis would be severe. Finally, one patient thought prognosis probably could be predicted by the doctors but did not have any idea what criteria were involved.

Question - What percentage of people with RA, ultimately, become completely disabled (i.e. unable to do most of the things necessary for self care)?

Patients' answers to this question are summarised in Table 6.11. As can be seen, most patients seem to be overestimating this risk - you will recall Huskisson and Hart (1978) report that less than 10% of people with RA become 'completely disabled'. The mean percentage suggested was 36.1% (median, 25; mode, 25). Two patients, in fact, thought that everybody with RA eventually becomes completely disabled.

Table 6.11

Patients' estimates of the risk of 'complete disability' as a result of RA

% completely disabled	No. suggesting this %
Over 60%	4
Between 30% and 50%	4
Between 10% and 29%	8
Less than 10%	1

Arguably a figure of less than 10% would be an underestimation for this sample, all of whom were rheumatology out-patients, but it is really rather difficult to say. Patients only get to see a rheumatologist if their G.P. refers them and G.P.s' knowledge and experience of RA, and hence, ability to recognise RA and the need for specialist care, is something that varies greatly - in a later study, reported in this book, involving 75 patients, it was notable that the same G.P.s' names kept cropping up. Additionally, those cases which present with the most dramatic symptoms, and as a consequence are quite likely to be referred, even by the 'reticent' G.P., are often among the less severe cases in terms of ultimate disability. Nearly half this sample had had their arthritis for five years or less and in most of these patients, although their disease was still fairly active and in that way quite disabling, obvious signs of permanent disability were not evident. Of patients with disease of longer duration, some did show quite definite signs of permanent disability and a couple had retired prematurely, but no patient was anything like completely disabled.

Duration of illness was not associated, at least not linearly, with patients' estimates of the risk of complete disability (rs=0.11, n.s.). However, among patients who have had their illness for some years, estimates of this risk do appear to reflect their own experience. The two patients who thought everybody with RA ultimately becomes completely disabled, had both been ill for many years and were probably the most, or at least, among the most, permanently disabled in the sample. Another patient, who had had RA for 33 years and reckoned the risk of complete disablement to be only 10%, was very much less disabled and very active physically. Patients who had been ill for less than five years all had fairly active disease and their estimates of the risk of disability appeared to be more independent of their own experience. Estimates among these patients ranged from 0% to 80%.

Question - What percentage of people with RA ultimately, have little or no disability?

Studies have shown that two thirds of patients with RA have minimal loss of function (Ragan, 1949; Duthie et al, 1964). More recently, Lorig and Fries (1980) report that 'only one in six persons with RA develops any crippling or deformities at all. And it is probable that these could have been prevented by good, early treatment' (p 8).

The answers of patients in this sample, to this question indicate that they underestimate the chance of remaining relatively unscathed from their arthritis (see Table 6.12). Even accepting the more conservative estimate of the consultant, that between 35% and 55% or RAs, ultimately, have little or no disability, all but one patient underestimated the likelihood of this outcome. The mean answer, based on the answers of 16 patients, was 15.55% (Median, 12.5; mode, 0). One patient would not commit himself to a percentage but commented 'not many' in answer to this question.

Table 6.12

Patients' estimates of the chance of, ultimately, sustaining no, or very little disability as a result of having RA

% little or no disability	No. of patients suggesting this
Between 20% and 50%	6
Between 10% and 20%	5
5% or less	5

Answers to this question did not correlate significantly with answers to the previous question (what percentage of people with RA, ultimately, are completely disabled) (rs=-.016, n.s.), or with duration of illness (rs=-.38, n.s.).

CONCLUSIONS

The knowledge of most of the patients in this sample about their condition and treatment was, to say the least, patchy. Only a few patients seemed to have anything like coherent and systematic information. The knowledge of most patients comprised odd snippets of information gleaned during consultations with doctors and from media coverage, but mostly was based on patients' own experience and deductions. It was not uncommon for patients to contradict themselves in the answers they gave to different questions. For example, one patient, in answer to the question about the disease process, said the joint fluid was depleted, but his explanation of swelling was that it was caused by an accumulation of fluid. Due to time restrictions it was not possible to try and resolve all seeming contradictions in patients' answers. Often attempts to resolve inconsistencies met with failure, reinforcing the impression that most patients had only a confused and incoherent understanding of their illness.

Consistent with the impressions gained in pilot study 1 was the tendency for patients in this sample to overestimate the risks of RA and underestimated the value of treatment. Although, contrary to this tendency, many patients seemed to underestimate the risk of drug side-effects and non-articular complications.

POSTAL QUESTIONNAIRE STUDY

Most of the open-ended knowledge assessment questions used in pilot study 2 were adapted for the questionnaire. Included were questions on prognosis, treatments and the disease process. For each question alternative statements or choices were selected from patients' answers in pilot study 2. Where necessary, additional alternatives were invented. As far as possible these invented alternatives comprised variations around common misconceptions about RA evinced in the pilot study. To enable the possibility of controlling for guessing, after each question patients were asked to indicate how certain of their answer they were by circling one of four responses, from 'totally or very uncertain' to 'totally or very certain'.

After removing a few questions which proved problematical, the remaining 29 item questionnaire (Figure 6.1) was distributed by post. In addition, patients were asked to record, on a separate sheet, any questions they had about RA.

Figure 6.1

Patient Knowledge Assessment Questionnaire Questions

1. Rheumatoid arthritis:
   1. Only affects the joints
   2. Only affects the joints and immediately surrounding tissues (e.g. muscles and tendons)
   3. Only affects the joints and blood
   4. Always affects the joints and can also affect many different organs and systems throughout the body
   5. Always affects the bones and in some cases also affects the blood and eyes but nothing else

2. Generally speaking, in RA exercise:
   1. Should be avoided as far as is possible because it wears the joints out more quickly
   2. Is good because it keeps you generally more healthy and fit and therefore better able to cope with a disease like rheumatoid arthritis
   3. Should be avoided as far as possible, as it makes inflamed joints that were previously alright

4. Is important as it helps, ultimately, to reduce the pain and inflammation
5. Is important, done correctly, as it maintains the movement and usefulness of the joint

3. The thing that most characterizes RA is:
   1. The inflammation or growth of the joint lining.
   2. The loss or drying-up of the joint fluid
   3. Chemical changes in the joint fluid (e.g. increased acidity or crystalization
   4. Loss of bone tissue
   5. Growth of abnormal bone

4. Some rheumatoid patients are given splints to wear at night which hold the hand and wrist in a set position. What do you think the main purpose of these splints is?
   1. To repair deformity
   2. To stop you lying on your hands and thereby stopping the blood getting to the joints
   3. To make your joints more comfortable through the night
   4. To prevent long-term deformities
   5. To hold the joints still so that they can be repaired overnight

5. When do you think it would be most important to wear night splints?
   1. When the joints are cool, not swollen or painful
   2. When the joints are very painful, swollen, hot and inflamed
   3. When you have not used those joints much during the day
   4. When you have used those joints alot during the day
   5. Every night is equally important, therefore, it does not matter when you wear them just so long as you wear them fairly often

6. RA most commonly stars:
   1. In childhood
   2. In adolescence (the teens)
   3. In early adulthood (under 25)
   4. Between the ages of 25 and 55
   5. In the over 55s

7. RA is:

   1. A chronic or long-term disorder
   2. An acute, or short-term disorder
   3. A disorder of intermediate length

8. What sort of exercise is best for the rheumatoid arthritic?

   1. Any sort of exercise done in moderation
   2. Exercises that put a strain or tension on the affected joints and thereby strengthen them (e.g. archery for the hand)
   3. No exercise is good - joints should be used as little as possible
   4. Exercises that involve quick jerky movements (e.g. squash, jogging)
   5. Exercises that put each joint through its full range of movement without putting a strain on the joints

9. Most of the pain experienced with RA is caused by:

   1. The acidity of the joint fluid eating into the joint tissues and bone
   2. The joint not having enough fluid to lubricate it
   3. The inflammatory process and the grinding together of bones.
   4. The joint fluid leaking into the muscle
   5. Sharp crystals that have formed in the joint damaging the joint tissues

10. Drugs used in the treatment of RA:

   1. Carry a low risk of side-effects (less than 5% of people on these drugs develop side-effects)
   2. Carry a fairly low risk of side-effects (around 5% to 10% of the people on these drugs develop side-effects)
   3. Carry a moderate risk of side-effects (10% to 20% of people on these drugs develop side-effects)
   4. Carry a fairly high risk of side-effects (around 20% to 50% of people on these drugs develop side-effects)
   5. Carry a very high risk of side-effects (over 50% of people on these drugs develop side-effects)

11. Deformity in RA is caused primarily by:

   1. Damage to the tendons and ligaments and loss of bone.
   2. Loss of muscle tissue

3. Abnormal growth and twisting or warping of the bones
4. Loss of muscle tone and strength
5. Loss of bone and abnormal bone growth

12. Ultimately in RA approximately what proportion of patients are completely disabled? (i.e. unable to do most of the things necessary for self-care)
    1. Over 70%
    2. Between 50% and 60%
    3. Between 30% and 50%
    4. Between 10% and 30%
    5. Less than 10%

13. Morning stiffness is produced by:
    1. The joint fluid gelling or getting more sticky or viscous overnight
    2. An accumulation of fluid in the joint tissues overnight
    3. A loss or reduction in the amount of joint fluid overnight
    4. The muscles involved in movement seizing-up due to inactivity
    5. The tendons and ligaments contracting or shrinking overnight

14. Which of these statements is true?
    1. There are two main categories of drug used in the treatment of RA - those which reduce the symptoms of pain and inflammation and those that also slow the disease down
    2. The only effect of drugs in the treatment of rheumatoid arthritis is to reduce the pain experienced
    3. There are drugs used in the treatment of rheumatoid arthritis which can actually cure the disease
    4. While there are drugs which actually reduce the symptoms of swelling and inflammation, as well as the pain, there are none which actually effect the eventual damage that rheumatoid arthritis does to the body
    5. All of the drugs used in the treatment of rheumatoid arthritis affect the speed with which the disease damages the joints

15. Ultimately in RA approximately what proportion of patients have little or no disability?

    1. Over 75%
    2. Between 55% and 75%
    3. Between 35% and 55%
    4. Between 15% and 35%
    5. Less than 15%

16. In RA, bone tissue:

    1. Turns to crystals at the outer edges
    2. Is not affected
    3. Is swollen or enlarged
    4. Is eroded or destroyed chemically and mechanically.
    5. Is first softened by joint fluid being absorbed into it and then crystalized by the chemical action of the joint fluid in the bones

17. Deformity in RA:

    1. Occurs in every case and cannot be prevented or lessened at all
    2. Is only avoided or lessened by the use of drugs
    3. Can only be avoided by stopping using the joint altogether
    4. Can probably only be avoided or lessened by adopting a very strenuous exercise programme
    5. Can probably be avoided, to some extent at least, by the careful use of the joints and the appropriate use of exercise and rest

18. In RA the amount of time that joints are very hot, inflamed and tender:

    1. Tends to increase with the length of illness
    2. Tends to lessen after a number of years and in some cases seems to stop altogether
    3. Tends to lessen after a number of years, but never stops altogether
    4. Does not alter with the duration of illness
    5. Tends to stay about the same or get worse

19. When a joint is very inflamed, tender and hot to what extent do you think, ideally, you should use or rest it? A hot inflamed joint:

1. Should be exercised as much as possible and ideally more than normal
2. Should be exercised very frequently throughout the day using special exercises that involve moving the joint fully without straining it
3. Should be rested completely except for moving it through its range of movement twice a day
4. Should be rested completely
5. Should be used as normal despite the pain

20. In RA, when a joint is hot, inflamed and very tender and painful, rest:

1. Makes you feel better but does not really help in any other way
2. Helps prevent long-term deformities, reduces damage to the joint, and helps reduce the hotness, inflammation and pain
3. Makes you feel better but actually makes long-term deformities and problems more likely than if the joint is used normally
4. Makes the hotness and inflammation stay longer than if the joint is used normally
5. Is bad as it makes the joint very stiff and reduces its mobility

21. In RA the joint membrane:

1. Becomes thinner and more delicate
2. Reduces in elasticity or stretch
3. Thickens, becomes inflamed and produces an abnormal tissue
4. Is eaten away and destroyed
5. Contracts or shrinks, reducing the space between the bones

22. In RA the joint fluid:

1. Is lost or decreased
2. Is crystalized
3. Is thinner and often increased
4. Gells or thickens
5. Is absorbed into the bones making them soft

23. In what way, if at all, is the way symptoms first occur predictive of outcome in RA?

1. An initial rapid onset of symptoms in many joints is associated with a more disabling arthritis
2. An initial rapid onset of symptoms in many joints is associated with a less disabling arthritis
3. A gradual onset of symptoms is associated with a less disabling arthritis
4. A gradual or slow onset of symptoms is associated with a more disabling arthritis
5. Type of onset of symptoms (rapid or gradual) is not associated with the degree of disability

24. It is possible to detect certain factors (rheumatoid factors) in the majority of cases of RA. These rheumatoid factors are:

1. A gene type (an inherited factor or unit)
2. Viruses (type of germ)
3. A type of blood cell
4. Joint fluid cells
5. Antibodies (a part of the bodies defense system)

25. High levels of rheumatoid factor in the blood:

1. Are associated with severe rheumatoid arthritis and more non-joint complications
2. Are associated with mild rheumatoid arthritis but more non-joint complications
3. Are associated with severe rheumatoid arthritis but less non-joint complications
4. Are associated with mild rheumatoid arthritis
5. Are not associated with the course of rheumatoid arthritis or frequency of non-joint complications

26. The cause of RA is:

1. Unknown
2. A virus (type of germ)
3. Genetic
4. The cold and damp
5. Wear and tear (the over use or bad use of the joints, accidents or old age)

27. Many patients are unsure about the amount of exercise to do. Which of these general guidelines do you think is correct?

   1. If after exercise your joints ache more than before the sort of exercise is wrong or you have overdone it
   2. Doing as much exercise as is possible, regardless of the effects afterwards, is best for the arthritis
   3. A level of exercise that does not make your joints ache more at all or makes then ache more for less than one hour is probably right
   4. A level of exercise that makes the joints ache more the next day, but no longer, is likely to do the joints most good
   5. No exercise is good for rheumatoid arthritis, whether it makes the joints ache more or not, therefore, it is important to keep exercise to the barest minimum

28. Rheumatoid arthritis:

   1. Occurs about twice as often in men as in women
   2. Occurs about twice as often in women as in men
   3. Occurs about ten times as often in men as in women
   4. Occurs about ten times as often in women as in men
   5. Occurs with equal frequency in both men and women

29. How common is RA? What percentage of the population has RA?

   1. About 2%
   2. About 10%
   3. About 25%
   4. About 40%
   5. About 55%

SUBJECTS

The sample receiving the questionnaire comprised every patient in the pool who had not yet been used (N=170, F=128, M=42).

The response rate was just over 77% - in total there were 128 (F=99, M=29) usable replies. The mean age of respondents was 55.7 (S.D. 10.41, median 58, mode 63) and mean duration of illness 18.7 years (S.D. 21.22, median 12, mode 6). There were no significant differences between respondents and non-respondents in age, male/female ratio, or duration of illness.

The questionnaire was sent to a second sample of patients (F=105, M=45) - all RA patients attending a rheumatology clinic in Torquay, a nearby town. A 76% response rate was obtained (F=79, M=35). Among respondents, mean age was 59.1 years (S.D. 12.88, median 62, mode 68) and mean duration of illness was 11.7 (S.D. 10.65, median 9, mode 1).

ANALYSIS AND RESULTS

Factor analysis of the questionnaire produced no reliable subscales of knowledge, although, solutions obtained were similar in both Exeter and Torquay patient samples. Coefficient alpha, for the final scale comprising 27 of the original 29 items, was .69 - two items with negative item-total correlations were removed.

In the pilot studies a tendency had been identified for patients to overestimate the risks associated with RA and, relatedly, underestimate the value of treatment. Eleven questions in the knowledge questionnaire allowed the expression of this 'negative bias', in so much as they presented alternative answers, more negative in implication than the correct answers (see Table 6.13). Consider, for example, question 12.

> Ultimately in RA approximately what proportion of patients are completely disabled (i.e. unable to do most of the things necessary for self-care)?
>
> 1. Over 70%
> 2. Between 50% and 60%
> 3. Between 30% and 50%
> 4. Between 10% and 30%
> 5. Less than 10%

The correct answer is alternative '5' - 'less than 10%'. Patients choosing any other answer are demonstrating 'negative bias'.

Table 6.13

Question and answer numbers of negative bias items.

Question Number	Answer Number(s)
2	1 , 3
4	2 , 3
8	3
10	4 , 5
12	1 , 2 , 3, 4
14	2 , 4
15	5
17	1 , 3
18	1 , 3 , 4 , 5
20	1 , 3 , 4 , 5
27	5

The 11 negative bias items (scored such that the selection of any negative bias alternative was coded as '1', while the selection of another incorrect alternative, or the correct answer, was coded as '0') did not scale, neither did factor analysis reveal any reliable negative bias scale.

(1) **Patients' Knowledge and Misconceptions about Rheumatoid Arthritis as Assessed by the Questionnaire**

The Mean knowledge score (27 item scale) obtained by the Exeter sample was 10.68 (S.D. 4.02, median 10, mode 10), the range of scores being from zero (N=2) to 23 (N=1). Among Torquay patients the mean score was 9.38 (S.D. 4.06, median 9, mode 9).

Knowledge score was not significantly associated with duration of illness ($r=-.086$, n.s.) but the number of questions asked about their condition did correlate significantly with knowledge score ($r=0.25$, $p<.02$).

Many of the misconceptions elicited in pilot study 2 were confirmed with this questionnaire. Tables 6.14 and 6.15 summarize various characteristics of the data. It can be seen for example that in 12 instances the single most popular answer was incorrect (Table 6.14).

Table 6.14

Percentage of patients choosing the correct and most popular incorrect answer to each knowledge question

Question No.	Correct answer	% choosing correct answer	Most popular incorrect answer	% choosing most popular incorrect answer
1	4	39	2	35
2	5	83	2	11
3	1	49	3	27
4	4	62	3	23
5	2	18	5	66
6	4	65	5	21
7	1	81	3	18
8	5	75	1	23
9	3	50	2	18
10	3	43	4	23
11	1	27	3	43
12	5	21	4	28
13	2	11	4	59
14	1	43	4	47
15	4	23	5	41
16	4	28	3	32
17	5	69	2	19
18	2	34	5	27
19	3	42	4	28
20	2	45	1	35
21	3	42	5	27
22	3	7	1	41
23	2	7	5	65
24	5	18	1 , 3	28
25	1	44	5	22
26	1	64	5	16
27	1	22	3	48
28	2	42	4 , 5	26
29	1	17	2	25

Table 6.15

Percentage of patients choosing a negative bias answer.

Question No.	Negative bias answer(s)	% choosing negative bias answer	% at least 'fairly certain' of negative bias answer
2	1, 3	4	2
4*	2, 3	25	20
8	3	2	2
10*	4, 5	34	20
12**	1, 2, 3, 4	79	23
14**	2, 4	53	41
15**	5	41	24
17	3, 1	10	6
18**	1, 3, 4, 5	66	45
20**	1, 3, 4, 5	55	33
27	5	19	13

* For these question a negative bias answer was the most popular incorrect answer.

** For these questions a negative bias answer was the most popular answer.

With regard to questions which allow an assessment of negative bias, with the exception of two (questions 2 and 8) - both concerned with the role of exercise - substantial proportions of patients chose a negative bias answer. This is the case even when only those patients saying they were at least 'fairly certain' of their response are considered (Table 6.15). For example 18% of patients were at least 'fairy certain' that splints only serve to 'make your joints more comfortable through the night' and a further 2% felt they merely 'stop you lying on your hands and thereby stopping the blood getting to the joints'. Similarly, 41% of patients were at least 'fairly certain' that the drugs available for RA only affected the pain (3%) or pain and inflammation (38%) but not the disease process, or its outcome. A total of 50% of the sample thought that at least 50% of people with RA ended up completely disabled. Twenty-seven percent of the sample were 'fairly certain' that the activity of the disease either increases or stays the same over the course of the disease; only 34% were aware that it sometimes stops and typically, gets less active over time. The significance of this negative bias and general illness knowledge, in terms of their affect on psychological distress and health behaviour, will be explored in later chapters.

(2) **The Questions Patients Asked**

Patients sent the questionnaire were also asked to note down any questions they had about their treatment or condition. Ninety-three patients (72.66%) asked at least one question and among those asking questions the mean number of questions asked was 3.71 (median 2, mode 2). The major type and sub-types of question asked are shown in Table 6.16, which gives the percentage of patients asking each category of question.

The most popular category of question was concerned with the treatment of RA, with patients being roughly equally interested in medical and self-help treatments. In particular patients were interested in the value of diet as a treatment (28%) and in the side-effects of drugs (29%), which together suggests than many patients, concerned about the side-effects of drugs, are interested in more benign alternatives.

Thirteen percent of patients were concerned that a particular symptom they were experiencing was a side-effect of a drug they were taking. In addition, 18% of patients were concerned to establish that a symptom they were experiencing was 'normal' or 'usual'. Thus quite a sizeable proportion of the sample were worried that a symptom they were experiencing was a sign of some problem additional to their arthritis. Most of the symptoms asked about are quite usual in RA (e.g. depression, tiredness, fever) - although a few of the side-effects were a little obscure - and suggests that a little simple information might alleviate some worry or at least indecision as to whether medical advice should be sought, pills discontinued etc..

The relatively high interest in self-help of all sorts also suggests a need for self determination and control - an issue which is recurrent throughout this volume.

Table 6.16

Percentage of patients asking different types of question

Question type	% asking this type of question (N=128)
ABOUT SYMPTOMS	32
-Is symptom usual?	18
-Why get symptom?	12
-What do about symptom?	6
ABOUT TREATMENT	61
-Self-help treatment	39
*diet	28
*exercise	10
*Unorthodox practitioners	10
-Medical treatment	41
*surgery	13
*drugs	37
+drug function	15
+side-effects	20
/specific	13
/general	5
ABOUT PROGNOSIS	23
ABOUT RESEARCH OR DISEASE PROCESS	23
ABOUT THE CAUSE	21
-hereditary	9
-idiosyncratic	9
COULD SOMETHING AFFECT THEIR ARTHRITIS	16
-climate	9
-stress	4

CHAPTER 7

METHODOLOGY OF THE MAIN CORRELATIONAL STUDY

Knowledge questionnaire data was supplemented for a sample of patients with data on health behaviour; emotional well-being and reactions to RA; and illness and personal details, gathered using an interview schedule and questionnaires during visits to their homes.

The methodology and analysis of this study is outlined here, while the main findings are discussed in the following three chapters.

SUBJECTS

Seventy-five patients were randomly selected from the original sample with the following provisos: that they lived within a 40 mile radius of Exeter; that the ratio of men and women who returned the questionnaire was preserved; and that they were not over the age of 75 years.

The patients interviewed had a mean age of 55 years, had suffered from arthritis for a mean of 15.6 years and had a mean knowledge score of 11.3. Socio-economic status was classified according to the Classification of Occupations and Coding Index (1980) and was based on present occupation or if a housewife or retired, on previous occupation. The composition of the sample in terms of occupation classification was as follows: group one, 0%; group two, 20%; group three (non-manual), 41.3%; group three (manual), 13.3%; group four, 17.3%; and group five, 6.7%. The mean age patients left school was 15.55 years.

INTERVIEW SCHEDULE

Patients were questioned about a number of topics:

COMPLIANCE

Practically it was possible to distinguish five different bimodal measures of compliance: current use of drugs, day splints and night splints; and whether patients had ever refused of dropped out of any drug treatment or non-drug treatment.

With regard to current drug use, patients were simply asked if they ever took more or less drugs than prescribed. As only three patients reported taking more drugs than prescribed compliers were simply compared with under users.

The assessment of compliance with splints was somewhat complicated by the variety of ways in which patients actually used their splints and by the fact that it seems likely that different patients had received different instructions. Splints are typically poorly tolerated and this is recognized by the occupational therapists (who provide patients with splints) who sometimes suggest compromises in their use such as, wearing a splint on the worst or most vulnerable hand, or in the case of day splints, using only for particularly heavy work. In view of these factors it was decided that any patient who indicated that they made a systematic and habitual attempt to use their splints, even if the way they used them was not quite as intended, should be classed as compliant, while patients who did not use their splints at all, or used them haphazardly (when the mood took them as it were), should be considered non-compliant.

USE OF UNORTHODOX TREATMENTS

Ss were asked if they had ever used or were using for their arthritis any of the following: heat; massage; prayer; faith healing; diet; dietary supplements; herbal or homeopathic remedies; topical applications; jewellery; or relaxation techniques. They were also asked if they had ever visited an unorthodox practitioner or made a trip for their health (e.g. visited Lourdes or another health spa). For each category of unorthodox treatment patients were prompted with a fairly comprehensive list of examples and then asked if they had 'tried anything else like that'. Each type of unorthodox treatment was also rated for 'helpfuless' using a seven point scale with end points labelled 'no help at all' and 'extremely helpful'.

EXERCISE HABITS

Patients were asked about the sort of exercise they undertook specifically for their arthritis.

MEDICAL TREATMENT

Patients were asked about their experience of RA drug side-effects. They were also asked to indicate on a four-point scale to what extent they minded taking drugs on a long-term basis. Their evaluation of the helpfulness of medical treatments was made on a seven-point scale with end points, 'no help at all' and 'extremely helpful'.

EMOTIONAL REACTIONS TO RHEUMATOID ARTHRITIS

Ss were asked to describe their emotional reactions to having RA and in particular were asked about periods of psychological distress. Additionally, patients were asked what good things, if any, had come out of their having arthritis.

DEMOGRAPHIC DETAILS AND ILLNESS HISTORY

Basic demographic details and illness history (age, occupation or last occupation, length of schooling, duration of illness) were taken.

QUESTIONNAIRES

BELIEFS ABOUT PAIN CONTROL QUESTIONNAIRE (BPCQ)

The BPCQ questionnaire (Skevington, in press) was used to assess patients' beliefs about control of their pain. The three scales of the questionnaire measure the extent to which people believe their pain is controlled by them personally (the internal scale - IPLC), is controlled by powerful others (the powerful others scale - PPLC) and is a matter of chance or fate (the chance scale - CPLC). Each comprises five statements with which patients indicate the extent to which they agree or disagree on a six point scale ranging from 'strongly disagree' to 'strongly agree'. Correlations among the subscales of the BPCQ are typically non-significant (Skevington, in press).

It was decided to use this questionnaire rather than the related Multidimensional Health Locus of Control Scale (Wallston et al, 1978) - the psychometric properties of which have been more extensively evaluated - as it was felt it would provide a more accurate assessment of patients' beliefs about control over their arthritis than the MHLC as pain is the most predominant symptom of RA and a good 'yardstick' of disease activity.

Skevington (in press) reports reliability coefficients for two small samples, one of chronic RAs and the other of undergraduates. For chronic RAs (retested 9.4 months later) correlations ranged from 0.53 for the chance subscale to 0.56 for the powerful others subscale. The coefficient for the questionnaire as a whole was 0.55. For the undergraduates (retested after a six week interval) the reliability coefficients range from 0.29 for the internal scale to 0.62 for the chance scale, with the coefficient for the questionnaire as a whole being 0.57.

Arguably as great interpersonal variation in pain is the norm in RA Cronbach's alpha (Cronbach, 1951) is likely to represent a more appropriate indicator of reliability. Reported alpha coefficients for the questionnaire range from .42 for a sample of acupuncture clients, to .91, for a sample of undergraduates. For chronic RA sufferers Cronbach's alpha is .72. Mean alpha, across six samples, is .63 (Skevington, in press). Skevington does not give alpha coefficients for the subscales, however, using the data obtained in this research (N=74) they are as follows: chance scale, alpha=.58; internal scale, alpha=.72; powerful others scale, alpha=.73.

Evidence of the validity of the BPCQ is provided by the finding of significant correlations between its subscales and those of related psychometric instruments (Skevington, in press), including the MHLC and Health Locus of Control scales. Notably, however, the internal scales of the BPLC and MHLC are negatively correlated.

GENERAL HEALTH QUESTIONNAIRE (GHQ-60)

The GHQ-60 is intended as a self-administered screening test of psychiatric disorder in the general population or community setting. Its items correspond to psychiatric symptoms or their inverse, and respondents are asked to compare their experience of each symptom 'over the past few weeks' with their 'usual' experience of the symptom. Although respondents indicate their answer on a four point scale the GHQ-60 is scored as a bimodal scale (no more than usual - more than usual) and, therefore, strictly speaking, represents a measure of change in psychiatric symptoms rather than an absolute measure; although in terms of case identification, the method of scoring (likert or bimodal) is reported as making little difference (Goldberg, 1978).

The recommended threshold score for distinguishing respondents with 'just significant clinical disturbance' is 11/12 on the GHQ-60. More specifically, Johnstone and Goldberg (1976) report that patients with scores between 12 and 19 tend to remit with time without treatment, while scorers of 20 or more only tend to improve if given treatment.

It is possible to extract from the GHQ-60 four subscales. In this study two subscales were used: the 'anxiety and insomnia' scale and the 'severe depression' scale . In the calculation of these scale scores items are scored 0-1-2-3 so that each subscale has a potential range of 0-21.

Split-half and test-retest reliability of the 60 item GHQ have been reported as being 0.95 and 0.75 respectively.

The GHQ-60 has been validated against two clinical interview assessment schedules - the modified Present State Examination (Wing, 1976) and the Clinical Interview Schedule (Goldberg et al, 1970). Correlation coefficients with clinical assessment range from 0.71 to 0.88. Evidence of construct validity is also available (Parker, 1975). Predictive validity coefficients for the depression and anxiety subscales have been reported as 0.56 and 0.71 respectively (Goldberg and Hillier, 1978).

A particular advantage of the GHQ-60 is that it was developed and validated on British samples and mainly on samples similar to the sample in this research (i.e. medical out-patients, and general practice patients). Its major drawback, in terms of this study, is that it asks about psychiatric symptomology in terms of variation from usual, and as such might be assumed to be insensitive to psychological distress occasioned by a physical illness of some duration. Indeed, there is some evidence to this effect (Goldberg, 1978; Barquero, 1982). However, others have suggested the GHQ-60 is appropriate for use with people with disorders of some duration. Pickering (1986) has suggested that respondents compare their present symptomology with what she describes as their 'personal concept of what is a normal state of being'. This is perhaps particularly likely to apply with a disorder like RA, which is marked by such great intrapersonal variability. Periods of relative remission of symptoms may serve to remind patients what a 'normal state of being' is like.

MCGILL PAIN QUESTIONNAIRE (MPQ)

The MPQ differentiates three major qualities of the pain experience - sensory, affective and evaluative. In addition it contains an intensity scale and a few other items relating to the pain experience (the miscellaneous scale). In the analyses detailed in this volume only the sensory and affective scales were used.

The sensory scale is comprised of 10 different subcategories of word, each subcategory concerned with a different type of sensory experience. Subcategory one, for example, contains six words which are concerned with temporal aspects of the pain sensation. The affective scale has five subcategories.

Within each subcategory the words are arranged in order of ascending intensity. Absolute intensity values, based on the judgements of doctors, patients and students (Melzack, 1975), can be assigned to each word and used to calculate a scale score or alternatively the intensity rank within each subcategory can be used. The correspondence between these two methods of scoring is very high and Melzack (1975) recommends the latter method in view of its ease of calculation - this method was used in the research reported here.

Self administration of the MPQ can produce unreliable data (Melzack, 1975) and, consequently, in this research, it was administered by the author, although, patients were given a copy of the questionnaire to follow.

Instructions to patients were that they should choose only one word from each subcategory but should only choose a word if it was appropriate. The only aberration from the method of administration prescribed by Melzack (1975) was to instruct patients to describe the pain they experienced most often rather than their present pain. Because the pain experienced in RA is so variable and is subject to diurnal variation, it was felt this change was necessary. Evidence that memory for pain is reliable using the MPQ is available (Hunter et al, 1979).

Judging the reliability of the MPQ is difficult. Test-retest reliability of the questionnaire might be expected to be low as pain tends to be quite variable. However, mean consistency of choice of subcategories has been reported as being 70.3% (Melzack, 1975) and 75% (Graham et al, 1980). Split-half reliability is also not very appropriate (and to date not reported) as different pain syndromes are best described by different subcategories of descriptor (Dubuisson and Melzack, 1976).

Face, construct, discriminant, and concurrent validity of the MPQ has been described as 'acceptable' (Reading, 1983). The questionnaire was actually developed on the basis of the judgements of a panel of judges but exploratory factor analytic studies of the questionnaire generally support Melzack's tripartite conceptualization of pain (see Prieto and Geisinger, 1983, for a review)

PAIN ASSESSMENT QUESTIONNAIRE (PAQ)

The PAQ, developed for this research, comprises three visual analogue pain scales. Each scale is 10cms long, with orthogonal end points labelled, 'no pain' and 'extremely severe pain'. The corresponding questions were as follows:

1. How bad is the pain that, LATELY, you have felt MOST OFTEN with your arthritis?
2. How bad is the WORST PAIN you have had with your arthritis over the PAST MONTH?
3. How bad is the LEAST PAIN you have been in at anytime over the PAST MONTH?

Patients were asked to mark the line at a point corresponding to the severity of their pain at these times. Care was taken to ensure patients understood the representation and what they had to do.

In scoring, the length of the line, from left to right, was taken to the nearest five millimetres. A measure of pain variability was computed by subtracting the score for scale three (least pain over the past month) from that of scale two (worst pain over the past month). Theoretically, this measure is of interest as predictability has been hypothesised as being the underlying dimension responsible for mediating the effects of feelings of control over the stress reaction (Thompson, 1981). It has also been suggested that RAs are particularly 'vulnerable' to unorthodox treatments because of the inherent disease variability of RA (see Chapter 4).

Test-retest reliability of visual analogue scales is generally found to be good - correlation coefficients as high as 0.99 have been reported (Scott and Huskisson, 1979).

Several studies indicate the predictive validity of visual analogue pain scales (Huskisson, 1976; Huskisson et al, 1979, 1980). Additionally,correlations between visual analogue measures of pain and other methods of assessment are good (Downie et al, 1978).

DISABILITY INDEX OF THE HEALTH ASSESSMENT QUESTIONNAIRE

Disability can be defined as the difficulty experienced in doing everyday activities such as washing, walking etc..

The Disability Index of the Health Assessment Questionnaire (HAQ) was specifically developed to assess disability in rheumatology patients (Fries et al, 1980). It is composed of eight categories, each of which has two or three component questions. The eight components of disability assessed are: dressing and grooming; arising; eating; walking; hygiene; reach; grip; and activities. Each question asks patients to indicate with how much difficulty they are able to perform various activities. Answers are given on a four point scale - without any difficulty; with some difficulty; with much difficulty; unable to do - scored, 0-3. If patients use devices to assist them or need the help of another person they are instructed to indicate the difficulty they experience when using the device or receiving assistance.

The score for each of the eight categories is the highest score obtained for any one of the component questions. If either devices and/or help from another person is indicated for a category the score is two, unless the score on any other component question is three. Total score, or disability index, is the sum of category scores divided by the number of categories answered. Principal components analysis supports the use of the scale as a unidimensional measure of disability (Fries et al, 1980).

Test-retest reliability of the HAQ is high. Measures taken six months apart have been reported as correlating as highly as 0.98 (Fries et al, 1982). Similarly, correlations of the scale with other scales (Brown et al, 1984) and with observer ratings (Fries et al, 1980) provide evidence of the validity of the HAQ.

STATISTICAL ANALYSES

Exploratory factor analysis was used as a method for organizing the associations between variables in a meaningful way.

Using SPSSX, principal components analysis was first computed and the scree test (Cattel, 1966) used to identify the optimum number of factors for extraction. Principal factors analysis was then performed and the solution rotated by Direct Oblimin (oblique rotation) to simple structure (Thurstone, 1947). Varimax rotation (orthogonal) was also computed as it was not clear which method of rotation would be most appropriate. As it turned out, Varimax and Direct Oblimin solutions were very similar but the oblique rotation produced the most meaningful and interpretable solution.

Two factor analyses were performed on the data. Table 7.1 shows the Direct Oblimin rotation, seven factor solution. In the analysis not shown the GHQ subscales of depression and anxiety were replaced with total GHQ-60 score. Two analyses were necessary in view of the fact that these subscales comprise items from the GHQ. Although they differed in terms of the number of factors identified (five and seven), fundamentally the two solutions were very similar.

The importance of the number of observations to variables ratio has frequently been discussed (see Nunally, 1978; Cattell, 1978; Barrett and

Kline, 1981). For most variables used in the factor analysis 74 or 75 observations were available. For three variables (non-compliance with night splint and day splint regimes; and use of drugs) considerably fewer observations were available (61, 50 and 65 respectively) simply because not all patients had splints or were taking drugs. As these variables were of particular interest they were included in the analyses and additional factor analyses computed excluding these three variables to check the solutions; the argument being that if the two solutions were basically different the reliability of the 'larger' solution should be considered dubious. In the event, the solutions were little changed, with the additional variables simply resulting in an additional factor concerned with compliance. Only the variable concerned with use of day splints was not included in the final depression/anxiety analysis as its inclusion was statistically problematical.

The significance levels of factor loadings was determined using the Burt-Banks (Burt and Banks, 1947) formula. According to this formula the size of the loading necessary to reach significance depends, among other things, on the factor number (see Table 7.1).

Table 7.1

Size of factor loading necessary to reach significance using the Burt-Banks formula

Factor	Factor loading
1	.233
2	.235
3	.236
4	.238
5	.24
6	.241
7	.243

A variety of other statistical analyses were used, including: the t-test, Mann Whitney U-test, chi square, analysis of variance, and regression.

Variables Key

ACUP	- Seen an acupuncturer
AFF	- 'Affect' scale of the MPQ
B	- Anxiety scale of GHQ
CHIRO	- Seen a chiropractor
CPLC	- 'chance' locus of control
D	- Depression scale of the GHQ
DNO	- Number of unorthodox diets tried.
DORDRUG	- Dropped out of or refused a drug treatment
DORNDRUG	- Dropped out of or refused a non-drug treatment
DRUGUSE	- Take less drugs than prescribed
DUR	- Duration of illness.
EXETYPE	- Do exercise for arthritis
FAITHH	- Seen a faith healer
GOODRATE	- Benefits accrued from illness
HAQ	- Disability scale of the HAQ
HBNO	- Number of 'herbal' remedies tried.
HNO	- Number of different ways applied heat to help with arthritis.
HOMEO	- Seen a homeopath
IPLC	- 'Internal' pain locus of control
J	- Used jewellery for their arthritis
M	- Used massage for their arthritis
MINDRUG	- Extent to which mind taking drugs
ONO	- Number of 'other/miscellaneous' unorthodox treatments tried
P	- Prayed about their arthritis
PAQ	- Typical pain intensity 'lately'.
PAVAR	- Pain variability
PPLC	- 'Powerful others' locus of control
RATEMED	- Rating of the helpfulness of medical treatment
RATEPSY	- Rating of the problem their emotional reactions to R.A. have represented
SCORE	- Illness knowledge score
SENS	- 'Sensory' scale of the MPQ
SES	- Socio-economic status
SESEXP	- Number of drug side-effects experienced
SPLINTN	- Non-compliance with night splint regimen

Table 7.2

Direct Oblimin rotation of principal factor analysis

	FACTOR 1	FACTOR 2	FACTOR 3	FACTOR 4
PAQ	.78098	-.00301	-.09444	-.06608
AFF	.76765	-.07187	.00801	-.10904
SENS	.67072	.10717	.07443	.00334
HAQ	.53399	.06395	.13021	-.08748
IPLC	-.24917	-.16227	-.22622	-.00711
RATEMED7	-.26574	.54036	-.21398	.10434
SCORE	.05648	.5191	.10854	-.05925
SES	.04219	-.40937	-.32341	-.00526
SESEXP	.02448	.40925	.11459	-.06465
ACUP	-.0741	-.38537	.12861	-.09356
EXETYPE	.15608	.38457	-.06024	-.25187
CHIRO	-.02583	-.36527	.11602	-.14446
DUR	.11242	.28703	-.0725	-.24736
DORNDRUG	.11064	-.02512	.62532	.09516
CPLC	.22422	-.35096	-.51856	.16732
DRUGUSE	.08157	-.09558	.51083	-.00058
PPLC	.1311	-.13509	-.35213	.26773
HBNO	.02467	.11461	-.01937	-.74963
ONO	.28116	.06519	-.0065	-.57809
J	.21642	-.02397	-.40835	-.41788
PAVAR	.18714	.20697	-.08166	.41122
DNO	.12274	-.15069	.00193	-.37883
SEX	-.09793	.05404	.05108	.24428
FAITHH	.18671	-.04209	-.2069	-.12284
AGE	-.0366	.05466	-.08552	-.06597
GOODRATE	-.15593	.22945	-.08452	.08349
P	.0819	-.18444	-.0453	-.21567
SPLINTN	-.05561	-.02669	.06667	.09399
M	.06467	.0903	-.21176	-.11809
DORDRUG	.1074	-.13929	.38871	-.19941
HOMEO	.00653	.05897	.04172	-.21414
HNO	.31888	.17138	-.11581	-.35824
B	.39569	-.06323	-.13946	.01688
RATEPSY	.16467	-.06037	.02788	-.22413
D	.18101	-.20969	-.23621	.27407
MINDRUG	-.00998	-.08723	-.00956	-.14094

Table 7.2 continued

	FACTOR 5	FACTOR 6	FACTOR 7
PAQ	.00535	.00204	.13064
AFF	-.15383	-.26186	.2747
SENS	-.0188	-.31263	.21175
HAQ	-.06678	.2897	-.126
IPLC	.15632	-.11511	.13329
RATEMED7	.22268	.17579	-.34209
SCORE	-.29512	-.11113	-.10126
SES	-.01882	.31283	.18652
SESEXP	.03577	.00002	.03477
ACUP	.07672	.18136	.20416
EXETYPE	-.08468	.15849	-.17902
CHIRO	-.20569	.02901	-.20603
DUR	-.00584	.07799	-.07961
DORNDRUG	.04875	.04716	-.03489
CPLC	.17462	-.12092	.28877
DRUGUSE	.22252	.12272	.0687
PPLC	.28942	.19677	.04586
HBNO	.01975	.02409	.13849
ONO	-.28848	-.13748	.16388
J	-.21663	.00365	.07103
PAVAR	.08946	.03199	.15562
DNO	-.2006	.1462	.20061
SEX	.62511	-.03513	-.01059
FAITHH	-.58216	-.07825	.05531
AGE	.52275	.07106	-.17885
GOODRATE	-.4255	.00307	-.22109
P	-.34762	-.11833	.2094
SPLINTN	.25782	-.11115	.22427
M	-.12495	-.45759	.06357
DORDRUG	.06151	-.44516	.15951
HOMEO	.00082	.40152	.14015
HNO	-.0487	-.36989	.28021
B	-.07808	-.07468	.78068
RATEPSY	-.17365	-.19945	.67203
D	-.19553	.0609	.48144
MINDRUG	.03208	.10373	.46365

Table 7.3

Factor correlation matrix

	FACTOR 1	FACTOR2	FACTOR3	FACTOR4	FACTOR5
FACTOR 1	1.				
FACTOR 2	.04008	1.			
FACTOR 3	-.02269	.00949	1.		
FACTOR 4	-.08205	-.02469	-.02393	1.	
FACTOR 5	-.09354	-.00286	.03096	.15044	1.
FACTOR 6	-.02352	-.02222	-.00596	-.00228	.0449
FACTOR 7	.14697	-.15678	-.04818	-.05373	.01949

	FACTOR 6	FACTOR 7
FACTOR 6	1.	
FACTOR 7	-.08299	1.

INTERPRETATION OF FACTORS

FACTOR ONE is clearly concerned with physical distress.

FACTOR TWO - high scorers on this factor are likely to rate their medical treatment highly, have a good understanding of their condition, a low chance pain locus of control score, be in a higher socio-economic group,and be less likely to have tried a chiropractor or acupuncturist. One interpretation of this factor is that it distinguishes patients who are satisfied with their medical treatment from those who are not. More specifically it may distinguish patients with a good relationship with their doctor from those without.

FACTOR THREE is concerned with non-compliance with conventional medical treatment.

FACTOR FOUR - loading most highly on this factor are those unorthodox treatments which patients choose and supervise themselves - such as over-the-counter herbal and homeopathic remedies, diets, jewellery and heat remedies.

FACTOR FIVE, if scored would tend to distinguish users and non-users of what might be termed intrapsyhic coping strategies - prayer, use of a faith healer, meditation, relaxation, positive reappraisal of negative events. Alternatively it may simply reflect religious faith.

FACTOR SIX - the interpretation of this factor is not as straightforward as the others. It seems likely this factor makes a distinction between patients with a preference for medication (homeopathy and medical drugs) and physical (e.g. heat, massage) treatments.

FACTOR SEVEN is concerned with psychological distress.

CHAPTER 8

PSYCHOLOGICAL DISTRESS - RESULTS AND DISCUSSION

INCIDENCE, SEVERITY AND NATURE OF PSYCHOLOGICAL DISTRESS

Using the recommended threshold of 11/12 for the 60 item GHQ (Goldberg, 1978), 31% of this sample, at the time of interview, could be described as having at least 'just significant clinical disturbance'. This is substantially higher than in general population samples (see Chapter 2) but substantially lower than the 53.5% point prevalence obtained in another sample of British RAs using the 30 item GHQ (Gardiner, 1980).

It has been reported that respondents with scores between 12 and 19 on the 60 item GHQ tend to remit with time, while those above 19 generally improve only if given treatment (Johnstone and Goldberg, 1976). In this sample 14.9% of respondents scored 20 or above. Mean score was 8.9 (range 0-40; S.D. 10.4).

Scores were calculated for the B (Anxiety and Insomnia) and D (Severe Depression) subscales of the GHQ. The mean scores for B was 5.6 (range 0-18; S.D. 4.2) and for D, 2 (range 0-13; S.D. 2.9).

In addition to the GHQ, patients were asked to rate, on a five point scale, the extent to which they felt their emotional reactions to having RA had represented a problem (Mean 2.7,range 1-5, S.D. 1.1). Also of relevance to the topic of this chapter, are patients' scores on the affect subscale of the MPQ (mean 2.7; range 1-10; S.D. 1.2).

Patients were also asked a series of open-ended questions about their emotional reactions to RA. Specifically, they were asked to describe feelings and emotions at times when they had been particularly distressed by their arthritis. A number of categories of response were identified from their replies. Details regarding the frequency with which each emotion was identified and whether it was described as being a current or past emotion are given in Table 8.1. Patients were also asked what it was about having RA that got them down (Table 8.2) and at what times or stages in their illness they experienced psychological distress as a result of having RA (Table 8.3).

Table 8.1

Qualitative nature of feelings and emotions experienced by patients at times of distress (N=75)

Emotional response	No. having felt this way	No. who still feel this way
Depressed	50	34
Frustrated	40	32
Tearful	36	19
Angry	31	22
Anxious	25	16
Desperate	17	1
Overwhelmed	12	10
Guilty	12	10
Suicidal	12	2
Embarrassed	4	4
Other	2	2

Table 8.2

Things about having RA that cause(d) distress.

Problem	No. mentioning this as a cause of distress	No. for whom this still causes distress
Disability/ restrictions	54	43
Pain	28	13
Hope/helplessness of situation	24	7
Fear of future	21	14
Reactions of others	14	11
Feel restrict loved ones	9	7
Fatigue	8	7
Deformity	8	8
Other	6	5

Table 8.3

Times or stages in their illness that patients reported being particularly distressed by their arthritis.

Time/stage	No. of patients	No. for whom this time is still bad
When restricted by arthritis	42	35
When arthritis is active	32	15
On and off (not tied to any specific time/ event)	26	25
Most of the time/ always	22	22
At first	21	3
When other things are going on/other life events	9	7
When there are new developments in arthritis	9	1
When arthritis prevents sleep at night	6	3
At diagnosis	3	-
Other	12	8

THE DIMENSIONALITY OF DISTRESS

Variables measuring psychological distress form a distinct factor (see Table 7.2). Other variables loading in the same factor as psychological distress include: the chance scale of the BPCQ (CPLC); rating of conventional medical treatment (RATEMED); number of different methods of applying heat tried (HNO); and the extent to which patients mind taking drugs on a long term basis (MINDRUG). These results are discussed in more detail below.

RELATIONSHIP OF ADJUSTMENT AND DEMOGRAPHIC VARIABLES

None of the demographic variables assessed (i.e. age, sex, and socio-economic status - SES) load on the 'psychological distress factor', and there exists just two significant correlations among these two sets of variables: SES is significantly correlated with depression (D) ($r=0.26$, $p<0.03$), and RATEPSY is associated with sex (point biserial correlation coefficient (r_{pb})$=-0.24$, $p<0.04$).

The association of SES and adjustment is consistent with previous research findings (see Chapter 2), and as in Brown's study (Brown and Harrison, 1978) can probably be explained by reduced 'coping resources' and increased life stress in the lower SES groups.

In our society there is a tendency for men to hide their feelings; the association of sex and RATEPSY may simply reflect this tendency. This result is also consistent with the suggestion, elaborated upon in Chapter 10, that men rely more on denial as a coping strategy.

The finding of one group of researchers that male RAs experience distress earlier in the course of their illness than women was not replicated in this study. Correlations between the three main adjustment variables (D, B, and GHQ) and illness duration revealed no significant differences for sex.

DISEASE VARIABLES AND ADJUSTMENT

Disease Severity

It is interesting to note that while anxiety is strongly associated with disease severity - it loads on the physical distress factor and is significantly correlated with all three measures of pain experience - depression is not associated with any measure of disease severity. More on this later.

The question of whether pain affects distress or vice versa clearly cannot be answered with this data. Theoretically, affect and pain are inextricably linked (Melzack and Wall, 1965).

Disease Duration

Disease duration (DUR) neither correlates with any measure of adjustment or loads on the psychological distress factor. The possibility that stages of adjustment, marked by distinct emotional responses, occurred was examined for depression, anxiety, tearfulness, guilt, frustration, anger and feeling overwhelmed, using chi square and analysis of variance - no analysis was significant.

CONTROL AND ADJUSTMENT

Chance pain locus of control (CPLC) beliefs are significantly associated with depression (D) ($r=0.35$, $p<0.003$), anxiety (B) ($r=0.26$, $p<0.03$), GHQ ($r=0.24$, $p<0.05$) and pain affect (AFF) ($r=0.29$, $p<0.02$), and CPLC loads on the psychological distress factor.

This pattern of results is consistent with the theory that the perception or expectation of non-contingency leads to psychological distress (Seligman, 1975; Abramson and Seligman, 1978). In line with this interpretation is the finding of a significant negative correlation between internal pain locus of control and AFF. Clearly, however, the possibility that the direction of causality is opposite to that suggested cannot be ruled out on the basis of this data.

Significantly, the finding that depression is associated with beliefs about control but not with the actual experience of pain or disability suggests, contrary to the predictions of the revised theory of learned helplessness (Abramson and Seligman, 1978), a direct effect of perceptions of control on distress.

The Health Locus of Control Typology and Adjustment

That the pattern of locus of control beliefs across the three scales may be more predictive of adjustment to illness than scores on any particular subscale was suggested by Wallston and Wallston, (1982). Specifically, it was suggested that 'believers in control' (Type V; high PPLC, high IPLC; low CPLC) or Type VII responders (high scores on all the subscales) would show better adjustment (see Chapter 2 for the reasoning underlying this hypothesis). The fact that CPLC is the only subscale to load on the psychological distress factor suggests that this typology aids little in understanding psychological distress in this population. This conclusion was confirmed using analysis of variance.

ILLNESS KNOWLEDGE AND ADJUSTMENT

Many of the worries and concerns expressed by patients in pilot study 1 seemed to be based on misconceptions about RA and reflected a general lack of information. The results of this study, however, do not support the idea that a lack of illness knowledge is contributing to psychological morbidity.

Illness Knowledge (SCORE) does not load on the psychological distress factor and is not associated with any measure of psychological distress. In regression of the other variables in the factor analysis on SCORE, only one variable, SES, achieved a significant beta weight (Beta=-.427; t=-.3.131; p<0.004; R squared=.182).

The possibility that a more clear-cut relationship between knowledge or beliefs and adjustment might emerge if a consideration of knowledge was restricted to those items specifically concerned with the evaluation of treatment and prognosis (Questions (Qs): 4, 10, 12, 14, 15, 17, 18, 20, and 27) was explored. The answers to these knowledge questions were ranked for optimism-pessimism (see Table 8.4) and regressed on GHQ, anxiety and depression. None proved to be a significant predictor of any measure of psychological distress.

Table 8.4

Coding of knowledge questionnaire items for pessimism

Question	Pessimism Rank (high=most pessimistic)				
	Answer No.				
	1	2	3	4	5
1	1	2	3	5	4
4	1	3	3	2	1
10	1	2	3	4	5
12	5	4	3	2	1
14	3	5	1	4	2
15	1	2	3	4	5
17	1	2	2	1	1
18	5	1	2	3	4
20	2	1	3	3	3
27	1	1	1	1	2

It seems feasible that the impact of illness knowledge on adjustment might depend, to some extent, on disease parameters such as duration and severity of illness; arguably, patients who have had their illness a long time or have only mild disease needing less information. This possibility was explored by comparing correlations between the three main adjustment variables (GHQ, B and D) and illness knowledge (using Fisher's Zr transformation) for patients in the top and bottom third of each of the following variable distributions: pain intensity (PAQ1), disability (HAQ), and illness duration (DUR). No significant differences were observed, however.

FEELINGS ABOUT CONVENTIONAL MEDICAL TREATMENT AND ADJUSTMENT

Two variables which tap feelings about treatment load on the psychological distress factor: the helpfulness of conventional medical treatment (RATEMED) and dislike of long-term drug use (MINDRUG). Both variables are significantly correlated with all the various measures of psychological distress (RATEPSY, GHQ, D, B, and AFF) with the exception that MINDRUG is not significantly associated with D.

RATEMED, as would be anticipated is positively associated with adjustment. The design of this study precludes any decision regarding the direction of causality of this effect, however, given the potential impact of a chronic disease like RA on one's life, one intuitively feels that feelings about treatment will affect distress.

The finding that RATEMED is significantly associated with psychological distress while beliefs about specific treatments is not appears somewhat contradictory. Notably, however, beliefs about the intended function and side-effects of specific treatments (coded for pessimism - see Table 8.4) are not significant predictors of RATEMED in regression. This may reflect the fact that patients' knowledge or beliefs about the treatment of RA in general do not necessarily reflect their beliefs about their own treatment. Or it may reflect the fact that many patients on disease modifiers do not know they are on them. Alternatively, it may be that patients rate treatments simply on the extent to which they can control their pain and whether treatments are supposed to modify the disease process, prevent deformity, or produce side-effects is largely immaterial - i.e the criterion on which they judge a treatment is short-term pain rather than long-term damage. Certainly all the measures of pain (SENS, AFF, PAQ1) are significantly associated with RATEMED.

Yet another interpretation is possible. Although not directly assessed, it seems likely that many patients, aware of the potential long-term benefits of treatments, judge their effectiveness in terms of immediated analgesia - an inappropriate guage. Thus many patients may erroneously be feeling that treatments do not work for them - a belief clearly likely to have a negative effect on psychological wellbeing. Statistically the effect of these unfulfilled expectations of treatment on wellbeing may be to counterbalance the positive effects experienced by patients more thoroughly informed.

The MINDRUG result suggests that fears about drug side-effects are contributing to patients' distress. That beliefs about the frequency of side-effects (Q10), and the number of side-effects actually experienced (SESEXP) are not associated with either MINDRUG or most measures of psychological distress suggests that a more likely explanation is that worrying about taking drugs and current psychological distress are concommitants of trait anxiety.

POSITIVE EFFECTS OF ILLNESS

Patients were asked if anything good had come from their illness and their answers coded on a four point scale ranging from zero (no good) to three (most good). Patients whose answers were coded as '3' typically indicated that their illness had caused them to re-evaluate their life or change their perspective on life in a positive way. The other most common responses were that their illness had brought them closer to their family (coded '2'), had made them more compassionate to other people (coded '1'), or had brought no benefits (coded '0'). Most people gave one of these answers in fact, although one or two gave others, such as one lady who said the only good to come from it was that it had caused her husband to finally leave (thus removing a source of great stress) and another who said that it meant she did not have to do housework (both these answers were coded '1'). A small number of patients gave more than one category of answer; in the factor analyses these were scored according to the highest category mentioned. In a few cases (N=6) this question was not asked as it was felt it would appear insensitive and give offence.

Table 8.5

Reported benefits of RA

Answer	% (N=68)
Nothing	51.5
compassion	20.6
Improved relationships	16.2
Personal growth	19.1

Clearly, the validity of the coding of this variable, GOODRATE, is questionable. However, some validation for the rank order imposed is provided by the fact that eight out of 10 'judges' confirmed it. The two that did not both felt compassion to be a greater benefit. The fact that patients who mentioned compassion seemed to have to search for something to say and made comments such as, '.. well I suppose it's made me more sympathetic to other people in a similar position', suggests that the used ordering is valid. Theoretically the ordering is consistent with Maslow's (1954) hierarchy of needs.

Interestingly, although GOODRATE is significantly associated with B (r=-0.23, p<0.05) it is not associated with any other measure of psychological distress and does not load on the psychological distress factor. This suggests that the ability to see something good, in what in many ways represents a devastatingly bad event, is distinct or independent from psychiatric adjustment.

In fact GOODRATE loads most highly on the 'faith' or 'intrapsychic coping' factor. The association of a 'personal growth' type of response and religious beliefs has been made before (e.g. Matson and Brooks, 1979). An appealing explanation for this finding is that, for some people at least, their faith helps them to see something positive in their illness. The likelihood that a person will both seek and see meaning in their illness is likely to be increased by a belief in an omnipotent and good God, especially if this leads them to believe their illness is God's will. Of course the inverse may also be true - the search for meaning may lead to a belief in God.

It may also be the case that the sort of 'mysticism' or 'spirituality' that favours religious faith , or more specifically use of faith healers - GOODRATE is only correlated with the use of a faith healer and not with personal prayer - also favours a positive interpretation of illness. Indeed, a variety of personality traits may account for the association (e.g. optimism, or open-mindedness). That GOODRATE is only associated with the use of a faith healer also suggests the idea of a religious experience or revelation rather than a gradual increase in reliance on religion and prayer. It may well be that faith healers help patients to see their illness as meaningful.

One other variable with which GOODRATE is associated, and which incidentally also loads on the faith factor, is age (r=-0.3, p<0.02). One interpretation of this result is in terms of the relative impact of a disabling condition like RA on the young and the old. Arguably, disease and disability is more disruptive and distressing in the young - certainly all the measures of psychological distress are negatively (although not quite significantly at the two-tailed level) associated with age. The association of GOODRATE and age may reflect the fact that only when a life event is very important and intrusive do we find it necessary to search for and, hence, find positive meaning for that event; in terms of Cognitive Dissonance theory (Festinger, 1975) only when dissonance is above a threshold do we make cognitive adjustments. Alternatively, the ability to see good in all things may be a characteristic of youth, perhaps one related to flexibility or innovativeness.

Certainly in addition to seeing it as an outcome variable, GOODRATE can itself be seen to be an intrapsychic or cognitive coping strategy in so much as it represents an attempt to reappraise loss as benefit. This interpretation seems particularly appropriate for patients experiencing a reorientation in perspective, for whom this issue seemed particularly salient.

SUMMARY

Patients reported experiencing a wide range of negative emotions because of their arthritis, including suicidal feelings, embarrassment, anger and guilt. Notably the most prevalent reported cause of distress was the restrictions arthritis imposed.

The pattern of correlations between the measures of anxiety and depression and other variables assessed in this research are fairly distinct. Anxiety is most strongly associated with pain while depression, which is uncorrelated with pain, correlates most strongly with chance locus of pain control beliefs and feelings about medical treatments.

Surprisingly, illness knowledge and specific beliefs about treatments and prognosis did not prove to be significant correlates of psychological distress, although patients' ratings of the helpfulness of their own medical treatment and concern about long-term drug use were both significant correlates of distress. However, before concluding that 'abstract knowledge', or beliefs about the function of treatments and prognosis, are of no psychological significance it is recommended that the hypothesis be retested once it is ensured that patients understand that the long-term efficacy of treatment cannot be accurately assessed in terms of short-term analgesia. Alternatively this variable might be controlled for statistically; unfortunately, with the present data set, this is not possible. If it transpires that this piece of information is a necessary prerequisite for benefitting from additional information about treatments then this would suggest it may be possible to identify a hierarchy of information provision for many illnesses.

CHAPTER 9

COMPLIANCE WITH CONVENTIONAL MEDICAL TREATMENT - RESULTS AND DISCUSSION

INCIDENCE OF NON-COMPLIANCE

Levels of non-compliance (see Tables 9.1 and 9.2) were fairly typical, although, possibly on the low side. The criteria of compliance used are outlined in the methodology chapter.

Table 9.1

Percentage of non-compliance with current treatments.

Treatment	% (N)
Night splints	32.8 (20)
Day splints	21.6 (11)
Drugs	13.8 (9)

Table 9.2

Percentage of patients refusing or dropping out of conventional medical treatment.

Treatment	% (N=74)
Drugs	21.6
Physiotherapy	14.9
Surgery	2.7
Other	1.3

The position of exercise as a conventional medical treatment is somewhat ambiguous in this study. Few patients actually reported being instructed to exercise for their arthritis, although, many reported having seen a physiotherapist (69%). Medically, however, exercise is generally considered appropriate and in this sample two thirds of the patients did exercise, to some extent, specifically for their arthritis. (The type of exercise done is shown in Table 9.3).

Table 9.3

Number of patients doing different types of exercise (N=50)

Exercises shown during physio-therapy	Other special exercises	Swimming	Other
31	17	3	10

THE DIMENSIONALITY OF COMPLIANCE

The factor solution indicate that compliance with conventional medical treatment (CMT) and use of unorthodox treatments, although both forms of 'illness behaviour', are independent behaviours. That compliance with different aspects of the regimen largely represent a single behavioural tendency is suggested by the loading of all but one of the compliance variables in the same factor (see Table 7.2). Use of day splints, which was not entered in this analysis for statistical reasons did load in the corresponding factor in the GHQ-60 solution (see Chapter 7). Other variables, all in fact loading negatively on this 'non-compliance factor', are: the powerful others (PPLC) and chance (CPLC) subscales of the BPCQ; socio-economic status (SES); use of jewellery (J); and depression (D). The association of compliance with these variables will be discussed in the following sections of this chapter.

Use of night splints (SPLINTN) does not load significantly with the other measures of compliance, and having dropped out or refused a drug treatment (variable DORDRUG), although loading significantly with the other measures of compliance, has its highest loading in another factor, one which seems to distinguish physical treatments (e.g. heat and massage) from drug treatments. SPLINTN, in fact, has its highest in factor five which appears to be concerned with reliance on faith in God as a means of coping with arthritis. Loading strongly on this faith factor is SEX and it seems likely that this accounts for the loading of SPLINTN on this factor - this hypothesis is discussed at length in a later section of this chapter.

PAIN LOCUS OF CONTROL AND COMPLIANCE

Both the powerful others (PPLC) and the chance (CPLC) subscales of the BPCQ load negatively on the non-compliance factor. Looking at the simple point biserial correlations, PPLC is associated with non-compliance with day splints (rpb=.25, $p<0.04$), and CPLC with refusing or dropping out of non-drug treatments (rpb=-.27, $p<0.02$). The predicted association of IPLC with those CMTs which involve self-control and discipline (i.e. exercise and splints) is not substantiated.

The association of PPLC and non-compliance is not very surprising and has been reported before (see Wallston and Wallston, 1982). The loading of CPLC on the non-compliance factor is more unusual. Wallston and Wallston (1982) report that chance beliefs are generally not found to be associated with compliance. A possible explanation for the association of CPLC and PPLC with compliance relates to the association of these variables and depression (see below).

The fact that the internal scale of the BPCQ does not load on the non-compliance factor suggests that the locus of control typology (described in Chapter 2) does not assist very much in understanding non-compliance.

PSYCHOLOGICAL ADJUSTMENT AND COMPLIANCE

The only measure of adjustment loading on the non-compliance factor is depression (D) - high scorers on this factor are likely to be less depressed than compliers. D is not significantly correlated with any one type of compliance, however.

While there is no reason to believe compliers are more depressed because their illness is actually more severe - no measure of physical distress (e.g. SENS, PAQ1, PAVAR, HAQ) loads on the non-compliance factor - it may be that they are more compliant because they are more psychologically distressed by their illness and thus, in a sense, more motivated. Arguably, the form of this distress, being depressive in nature, lends itself more to compliance with the advice of others than self-instigated activity - use of self-supervised unorthodox treatments is in fact negatively associated with D (see next chapter) - as associated with depression are feelings of personal inadequacy and impotence; apathy (motivational deficit); and a cognitive deficit or bias which enhances feelings of personal helplessness. Alternatively, in some cases compliance may simply reflect this apathy. In many respects, given the social pressure to comply (Parsons,1951), compliance is simply the easiest thing to do. The loading of PPLC and CPLC on the non-compliance factor supports these interpretations.

DEMOGRAPHIC VARIABLES AND COMPLIANCE

Socio-economic Status

The only demographic variable loading significantly on the non-compliance factor is socio-economic status (SES). This result indicates that non-compliance in this sample is greatest in the higher socio-economic groups. SES is not correlated with compliance with any particular treatment.

A likely explanation for this finding is in terms of the nature and quality of the doctor-patient relationship, and patients' beliefs about and reliance on powerful others. Patients from the higher socio-economic groups, because of their education and background, are likely to be more selective, evaluative, and discriminating regarding their treatment. Additionally, where the status and cultural gap between doctor and patient is small or non-existent, a style of interaction that Szasz and Hollander (1956) refer to as 'mutual participation' is more likely to occur (Hauser, 1981). In this type of doctor-patient relationship the doctor fulfills the role of 'professional advisor', but is not the dominant member of the dyad. His role is to set out the treatment alternatives, stating the 'pros' and 'cons' for each, and with the patient resclve on the most suitable treatment. There is no obligation on the part of the patient to accept any treatment or to stay in treatment if it is found to be unsuitable.

The doctor-patient relationship was not directly assessed in this study, hence, it is not possible to say to what extent it accounts for the relationship of SES and compliance. However, SES does load on factor two and one interpretation of this factor is that it reflects the quality of the doctor-patient relationship.

Age

The finding that younger patients are more likely to be non-compliant with day splints (rpb=-.29, p<0=.02) is probably largely explained by the tendency for older patients to have stronger beliefs in powerful others (rpb=0.35, p<0.003), but may also reflect the fact that the visibility and unattractiveness of day splints is particularly off-putting for younger patients, in whom disability is more unusual and, consequently, embarrassing. This self-consciousness was highlighted by one young woman who told of the embarrassment of having to be helped by her husband on the beach - the incongruity between her agility and her age she felt made her a particularly interesting 'spectacle' for other people on the beach. Many other patients commented that they hated people noticing and expressing sympathy about their arthritis and one relatively young patient (39 years) actually reported that she never wore her splints out as she felt too self-conscious.

Sex

Sex does not load on the non-compliance factor but it is associated with use of night splints and these two variables both have their highest loadings in factor five. Gender is not significantly associated with any other measure of compliance, although, the tendency is for men to be less compliant (see Tables 9.4 and 9.5). The only contrary results relate to the use of day splints and past refusal of drugs. However, in the latter case the rates of non-compliance for men and women differ by only two percent and in the case of day splints the higher compliance rate among the men may reflect a selection bias of sorts; men are less likely than women to have day splints (this result almost reaches significance, see Table 9.6). This bias may be due to the men refusing the idea or offer of day splints or may be due to preselection by medical staff. In fact, men are also less likely to have night splints or to be on drugs than women (see Table 9.6) and comparing subjects using their drugs and night splints correctly with those who are not on these treatments or use them incorrectly, (see Table 9.7) men are less reliant on drugs (this result approaches significance at the two-tailed level) and significantly less likely to be using night splints correctly.

Table 9.4

Percentage of patients complying with current treatments, shown separately for men and women

Type of treatment	Men %	Women %	Chi square
Night splints	33.3	62.7	5.98*
Day splints	85.7	76.7	0.00
Drugs	69.2	90.4	2.33
Exercise	56.2	69.5	0.49

* p<0.02

Table 9.5

Percentage of patients refusing or dropping out of treatments, shown separately for men and women.

Type of treatment	Men %	Women %	Chi square
Drug	20	22	0.00 n.s.
Other	26.6	16.9	0.2 n.s.

Table 9.6

Percentage of patients on treatments (i.e. in a position to comply), shown separately for men and women

Type of treatment	Men %	Women %	Chi square
Night splints	75	83	0.14
Day splints	43.7	72.9	3.58*
Drugs	81.2	88.1	0.25

* p<0.10

Table 9.7

Percentage of patients using treatments correctly, shown separately for men and women.

Type of treatment	Men %	Women %	Chi square
Drugs	56.2	79.7	2.97*
Night splints	25	62.7	5.78**
Day splints	37.5	55.9	1.05

* $p<0.10$, ** $p<0.02$

Night splints are, by all accounts, not the most comfortable or convenient of contraptions and are not conducive to an undisturbed night's sleep. Many patients commented that when they wore splints they woke up after a couple of hours because they were rubbing, or made it too difficult and uncomfortable to turn over in bed. Others mentioned that they felt helpless and dependent strapped into their night splints; two splints could only be worn if someone helped them into them and if two were worn patients could only use the lavatory in the night, or for that matter do anything but sleep, if they first woke their partner to 'free them'. Apart from the discomfort and the danger of incapacity, night splints, on some wrists, also represent a hazard for spouses. One lady remarked that her husband 'forbade' her to wear them after an incident where she had 'clunked' him in the face with one in the middle of the night.

It may be that the men in this sample, or their spouses, were simply less tolerant of this discomfort and inconvenience. It may also be the case that men, because of their relatively higher status in our society, feel less compunction to comply with a treatment in such circumstances. Alternative interpretations for the relationship between sex and health behaviour in general, as opposed to just the use of splints, are discussed in Chapter 10 as gender is more strongly related to the use of unorthodox treatments than CMTs. At this juncture suffice it to say that the interpretation favoured by this author is that the male reticence in practising health behaviour in this sample reflects their greater use of denial as a coping strategy and the need to preserve their 'manly image' - concern with health behaviour is considered effeminate. (The reasoning and evidence behind these assertions is presented in Chapter 10).

ILLNESS KNOWLEDGE, HEALTH BELIEFS AND COMPLIANCE

None of the measures of compliance are associated with illness knowledge (SCORE) and knowledge does not load on the non-compliance factor.

This result is not very surprising, measures such as SCORE, which assess fairly general knowledge about illness, have typically not been found to be associated with compliance in the literature (see Chapter 3). More specific knowledge or beliefs about treatment regimens (e.g. what to do and why) have, however, been found to be fairly consistently related to compliance. One of the aims of this research was to compare the predictive value of general and specific knowledge in the same study.

From pilot study 1 came the suggestion that some patients were underestimating the intended function or value of their treatment (this was confirmed by pilot study 2 and the knowledge questionnaire data) and this it was felt was leading to increased rates of non-compliance. Analyses looking at the relationship of compliance and patients' answers to knowledge questionnaire items concerned specifically with the function of treatments provide only weak support for this hypothesis, however.

Quite definitely in support of the hypothesis was the finding that patients' beliefs about the function of splints (question (Q) 4) was associated with their use of night splints; patients who underestimated the function of splints being significantly less likely to use them (chi square=4.65, $p<0.05$). Not quite significant at the two-tailed level was the finding that patients who felt exercise was bad for RA were less likely to exercise (chi squared=3.41, $p<0.07$). Similarly, although in the right direction, patients who underestimated the function of drugs (Q14) were not significantly more likely to use less drugs than prescribed (chi squared=0.17, n.s.) nor were they more likely to have dropped out of or refused drug treatments in the past (chi squared=0.27, n.s.); and beliefs about the function of splints was not associated with use of day splints (chi square=0.06, n.s.).

For questions 4 and 14 the small number of patients overestimating the function of treatments (five and two respectively), in conjunction with the relatively low levels of non-compliance, precluded a consideration of the effects of overestimating the function of treatments on compliance using chi square analyses. However, for both these questions the five alternative answers were ranked for optimism-pessimism (see Table 8.4) and the above comparisons repeated using the Mann Whitney U-test. The pattern of significant results was unchanged. As before beliefs about the function of splints (Q4) distinguished compliers and non-compliers with night splints (z=-2.16, p<0.04) but not with day splints (z=-1.95, n.s.). Beliefs about the function of arthritis drugs (Q14) did not distinguish compliers and non-compliers with current (z=-0.22, n.s.) or past advice (z=-0.31, n.s.) regarding medications.

Beliefs about the function of treatments represents just one component of the Health Belief Model (HBM) (see Chapter 3). Additionally, according to the model, other considerations will affect the subjective value or 'net benefit' of treatment and, hence, compliance. In this research patients' beliefs about the side-effects of drugs and the inherent risks of RA might be expected to predict compliance.

Q10 of the knowledge questionnaire assessed patients' beliefs about the probability of experiencing side-effects on arthritis drugs - answers 1-5 represent an ordinal increase in perceived risk. A Mann-Whitney U-test reveals that, contrary to the predictions of the HBM, people who believe the risks of side-effects are relatively high are no more likely to take fewer drugs than prescribed (z=-1.77, n.s.). Similarly, the extent to which patients report minding taking drugs (MINDRUG), and the number of drug side-effects they had actually experienced, are not related to use of drugs or to beliefs about the frequency of side-effects.

Beliefs or knowledge about the severity of arthritis were assessed by five questions (Qs 1, 12, 15, and 18) in the knowledge questionnaire. For each question it is possible to rank the five answers on a five point scale representing an ordinal increase in pessimism regarding prognosis (see Table 8.4). A series of Mann Whitney U-test analyses revealed that only two questions, coded for pessimism, distinguished compliers and non-compliers. People who had refused non-drug treatments in the past (DORNDRUG) were more likely to be aware of the wide ranging effects of RA (Q1) (z=-2.28; p<0.03). This result is contrary to the predictions of the HBM concerning beliefs about severity, but is consistent with the idea that feelings of hopelessness predispose to non-compliance. Also inconsistent with the HBM was the finding that the smaller the percentage of RAs patients felt ultimately had little or no disability the less likely they were to use their night splints (z=-2.31, p<0.03).

Finally, the main 'negative bias' questions (Qs 4, 10, 12, 14, 15, 18, 20, 17, 27) and Q1, ranked for pessimism (high rank=most pessimistic, see Table 8.4), were regressed (stepwise), on a computed non-compliance score (the unweighted sum of non-compliance variables in the non-compliance factor - alpha=.6). Only two questions obtained significant beta weights, Q12 (Beta=0.286; t=2.55, p<0.02) and Q4 (beta=-.279; t=-2.498, P<0.02) (R squared= 0.162). Again both these results are contrary to the predictions of the HBM; Q12 being concerned with patients beliefs about the chances of becoming completely disabled and Q4 being concerned with beliefs about the function of splints.

The lack of support for the HBM may reflect the fact that general beliefs or knowledge about RA do not reflect patients' beliefs about their own prognosis and treatment. Some indication that this is the case is provided by the finding, first reported in the previous chapter, that patients' beliefs about the intended value or function of specific treatments (Qs 4, 27, and 14 of the knowledge questionnaire) are not significant predictors of RATEMED.

It is also possible that the predictions of the HBM were not borne out because of the presence of an overriding negative bias in beliefs. In terms of the HBM the effects of overestimating the risks of RA and underestimating the benefits of treatment on compliance are opposite, and therefore, are likely to cancel each other out. The only problem with this interpretation is the fact that 'negative bias' beliefs did not scale very convincingly, suggesting that the tendency to hold one negative belief is not particularly strongly associated with the tendency to hold any other.

SUMMARY

Contrary to expectations the factor analysis indicated that compliance with different components of the regimen in this sample of RAs represents a general behavioural tendency and notably, one distinct from unorthodox treatment use.

The pattern of factor loadings suggests that to some extent at least this behavioural tendency is characterised by subservience, or at least, unassertiveness. Patients who do as they are told and take what they are offered tend to be of lower socio-economic status and feel more depressed and less in control of their illness than non-compliers. They are also more likely to be women. An alternative interpretation for the association of sex and compliance, however, is that men find the admission of weakness inherent in the acceptance of treatment less tolerable than women.

CHAPTER 10

USE OF UNORTHODOX TREATMENTS - RESULTS AND DISCUSSION

AMOUNT AND TYPE OF USE

To facilitate analysis some preliminary categorization of unorthodox treatments (UTs) was necessary. The major categories distinguished were: heat; massage; non-prescribed herbal/homeopathic remedies and dietary supplements (hereafter, referred to as herbal remedies); diets; prayer; jewellery; and alternative practitioners. Table 10.1 shows the number of patients having tried and at interview currently using each of the major types of UT distinguished. Patients' mean helfulness rating (7 point scale) for each type of treatment is also shown.

Table 10.1

Number of patients having tried and currently using each category of UT.

Unorthodox treatment	No. having tried this treatment (No. currently using)	Mean Rating
Heat	68 (44)	4.5
Massage	37 (35)	4.5
Herbs	52 (25)	2.7
Prayer	46 (41)	4.6
Diet	37 (75)	3.8
Practitioner	48 (10)	3.3
-chiropractor	14	4
-faith healer	25	2.3
-acupuncturist	15	4
-homeopath	9	2.1
Jewellery	46 (3)	1.6
Other	32 (21)	4.1

In line with Kronenfeld and Wasner's (1982) findings, slightly under 95% of patients had tried an UT, of one sort or another, for their arthritis. Indeed, most patients had tried several and one patient reported trying 20. The mean number of UTs tried was 5.85. Most patients were trying at least one UT at the time of interview - only 12 were not and the mean number being used at the time of interview was 1.9. If one includes the use of heat (variously applied) and massage as UTs then only one patient had tried nothing and was presently using nothing and the mean number of UTs tried is increased to 8.6, with the mean number of treatments being used at interview being 3.8.

Heat/Cold

The application of heat and cold to affected joints is actually undertaken in physiotherapy and recommended for home use in some instances, hence, it is not strictly speaking an UT. However, most patients seemed to have taken the decision to use heat themselves, unguided by the medical profession, and this self initiation it shares in common with other UTs, hence, its consideration in this chapter.

In terms of the Gate Theory of pain (Melzack and Wall, 1965) the application of heat or cold will reduce the intensity of pain experienced because it stimulates the large A-beta fibres which serves to inhibit, at the spinal cord, the transmission of the pain impulse to the brain. In addition, the application of cold will serve to reduce the inflammation.

Methods of applying heat were various and included: hot water bottles; heated pads; electric blankets; hot baths, showers, and basins of hot water for hands and feet; embrocations; poultices; heat lamps; sun lamps; sitting in the sun; extra layers of clothing; and sitting by the fire. Over 60% of patients had tried more that one method. Cold, on the other hand, was seldom used and most patients were fairly aghast at the thought.

Massage

Physiologically, massage is likely to have a similar effect as heat but is unlikely to be used on a very inflamed joint which is likely to be too tender to touch.

Where patients massaged things in, care was taken to elicit whether that patient actually believed the massage part to be independently important and the data coded accordingly.

Over the Counter Herbal Remedies

This was the second most popular type of UT tried and among those people trying at least one, the mean number tried was 3.4 (2.3 overall). Most of the remedies of this type were obtained from health food shops. Again the variety of remedies was considerable. Among the more popular were: cider vinegar, garlic pearls, ginseng, celery seeds, cod liver oil, feverfew, and biochemical salts.

The popularity of this type of remedy probably reflects its ease of administration and availability. That patients were a little disillusioned by such remedies is suggested by the fact that over half the people who had tried one were no longer using one.

It was felt the summing of these different remedies prior to factor analysis was valid for a number of reasons. First, most people who had tried this type of remedy at all had tried more than one specific remedy, and all involved taking pills or 'medications' and there is already evidence which suggests a 'pill taking type' (Pickering, 1986). Secondly, the absolute number of different remedies taken necessitated some grouping together and alternative groupings (e.g. dietary supplements vs herbal remedies vs homeopathic remedies) although theoretically sensible, in practice did not seem so as in their marketing these distinctions were not really made. It seems that while health food shops are allowed to sell dietary supplements they are not allowed to sell 'medicines'; hence, everything tends to be labelled as a dietary supplement. That patients tended to lump all these remedies together is indicated by the fact that while asked separately about their use of herbal/homeopathic and dietary supplements, they very often confused the two, primarily reporting their use of dietary supplements when asked about herbal/homeopathic remedies - the preceding question.

Diets

Some patients had adopted strict arthritis diets, whereas others had merely adopted certain dietary guidelines. The most common recommendations were: the exclusion or reduction of red meats, 'acid foods', dairy products, and additives from the diet; and an increase in fish, vegetables and whole grain products. Some diets included all these recommendations, while others made just one or two.

As with most UTs, much of the evidence supporting the use of special diets for arthritis involves case studies. However, recently their has been some medical research on the use of diet in the treatment of RA (Kremer et al, 1985), and the preliminary conclusions of this research is that diet may help some suffers. Specifically, polyunsaturated fat is thought to be of benefit.

Jewellery

Only three patients currently wore jewellery, such as copper bracelets and rings, for their RA, although, over 60% had at some time tried it. The most common comment regarding the use of copper jewellery was that they had worn it until it turned their wrist black! A few people reported persevering with it for a year or more, but typically it was tried for a few months and sometimes less.

The pattern of use suggests that its accessibility (both in terms of knowledge about it and ease of actually obtaining it) made it a remedy that was tried early in the illness and fairly quickly dismissed as gimmicky.

Unorthodox Practitioners

Considering the expense, it is perhaps surprising that so many patients had tried an unorthodox practitioner of some sort and quite a few had seen more than one (Mean 1.58, amongst users, range 1-6). However, only 10 patients were actually attending an unorthodox practitioner at the time of interview, and most patients who had attended one had done so for only a short time.

As it seemed likely that the reasons people seek unorthodox practitioners would vary according to the type of unorthodox practitioner it was decided to enter the different types separately into the factor analysis. However, due to the relatively small number of patients using some types of practitioner, and the relatively high 'competition' amongst variables for a place in the factor analysis, only the four most popular types of unorthodox practitioner were entered. Those not included were the masseur, dietitian, naturopath and allergist, seen by five, two, one, and one patients respectively.

Other Types of Unorthodox Treatment Used

Patients had tried a variety of other UTs, including trips to health spas and hotter climes; relaxation techniques; breathing exercises; yoga; meditation; oil rubs; reflexology; 'talking to joints'; bath salts; and even putting nutmeg in their socks.

THE REASONS PATIENTS GAVE FOR TRYING UNORTHODOX TREATMENTS

Patients were asked what had motivated them to try UTs. The most popular answer was 'desperation' (N=23). Basically, these patients implied they had tried UTs as a 'last resort' when things were bad and, clearly, because modern medicine was not containing their symptoms adequately.

The second most frequent answer suggested the use of UTs as an optimizing strategy (N=19). The sort of comments such patients made were along the lines, '.. I thought why not', '.. it might do some good and can't do any harm', and '.. I'll give anything a go'.

For quite a few people the motivation to try UTs was not really their own. As suggested in Chapter 4 many people are aware of UTs and keen to recommend them. Eighteen patients said they had been persuaded to try an UT by somebody else. Very often such patients were men and the people recommending, and often actually obtaining or arranging the treatments, their wives or daughters.

Surprisingly, only five patients implied they had been searching for a real alternative to modern medicine. Such patients were concerned about the side-effects associated with conventional medical treatment (CMT). This may be an underestimation of the frequency of this motive as patients may have been reticent about stating this reason to me who they may have seen as being a representative of conventional medicine, having been introduced by a letter from the consultant.

Most patients gave only one reason why they had tried UTs and did not distinguish different reasons for different treatments. However, as with most behaviours, use of UTs is in most cases probably multi-determined. In the following sections the pattern of associations among the different UTs and between UTs and a variety of other variables will be considered.

THE DIMENSIONALITY OF UNORTHODOX TREATMENT USE

The factor solutions suggest that the tendency to use UTs is not unidimensional. The different UTs have their highest loadings in four distinct factors.

Factor four is dominated by those UTs which patients choose and supervise for themselves (e.g. over-the- counter herbal remedies, jewellery, diets, heat)- hereafter referred to as self supervised UTs (SSUTs).

Loading significantly on factor five is use of prayer and the faith healer. Also loading on this factor, but not quite so highly, is 'miscellaneous' UTs. The loading of this last variable is consistent with an interpretation of this factor as being concerned with religious faith or what might be described as spiritually oriented or intrapsychic treatments. Among the 'miscellaneous' UTs tried were trips to health spas (e.g. Lourdes), meditation, relaxation techniques, and Yoga, activities all of which can be seen to have a certain spiritual significance. Another variable loading significantly on this factor is GOODRATE, which is consistent with the above interpretation of this factor.

The factor on which acupuncture and chiropractor use load most highly appears to be concerned with patients' feelings about CMT; with variables such as RATEMED, knowledge about RA, number of side-effects experienced, and whether patients mind taking drugs on a long-term basis loading on it. One possible interpretation of this factor is that it is concerned with the quality of the doctor-patient relationship, although, this was not actually directly assessed in this research.

Finally, massage, use of a homeopath and heat have their highest loadings in a factor which, if scored, would probably best distinguish users of physical of external treatments (e.g. massage and heat) from 'pill-takers'.

The pattern of factor loadings and simple associations between UTs and other variables will be considered in more detail below. The results are discussed under headings corresponding to some of the major hypotheses evident in the literature and developed in this book (see Chapter 4) concerning UT use.

DISEASE VARIABLES AND UNORTHODOX TREATMENT USE

Disease Severity

Although several of the UTs are positively associated with the pain affect scale (AFF) of the McGill Pain Questionnaire (MPQ) - which taps patients' emotional reactions to their pain - assessment of pain intensity using a visual analogue scale (PAQ) and the sensory scale (SENS) of the MPQ are only associated with the use of heat and massage. As both of these treatments are likely to be particularly effective in dealing with the sensory experience of pain this result is quite sensible. Disability (HAQ) is not correlated with the use of any one UT but loads with the pain variables, massage and use of heat on factor six. This result probably reflects the positive association between pain and disability.

Disease Variability

The suggestion that RAs are particularly liable to turn to UTs because of the inherent intrapersonal variability of the disease is not substantiated by this research. Disease variability, or more correctly pain variability (PAVAR), does load on the 'SSUTs factor' but in the opposite direction to that predicted by this hypothesis. It is of course possible that had the analysis contained other measures of UT use (such as length of use) and disease variability (e.g. frequency of change rather than magnitude of variability), and/or involved data from people suffering from a variety of illnesses (varying in terms of their mean intra-individual variablility) that this hypothesis would have been supported. Arguably, in the absence of variability, which according to this hypothesis allows the illusion of control, the search for control continues, hence, the result that greater use of UTs is related to low variability. This interpretation seems unlikely, however, as in this data set, pain variability correlates positively, albeit not quite significantly at the two-tailed level, with chance locus of control ($r=.214$, $p<0.07$), suggesting that, if anything, the intrapersonal variability of the disease fosters feelings of no control or helplessness.

An alternative interpretation is that high disease variability results in feelings of helplessness and a consequent lack in initiative and motivation, and, hence, less trying of UTs - this is in line with the Learned Helplessness Theory of depression (Seligman, 1975). Supporting this interpretation is the fact that PAVAR and depression load together on the factor concerned with SSUT use.

It is of course possible that the use of UTs actually results in a reduction in disease variability (i.e. achieves its aim of control), or at least this perception. The extent to which this is the case cannot be answered by this research except to say that, on the whole, patients do not rate UTs very highly (see Table 10.1 of this chapter).

PSYCHOLOGICAL DISTRESS AND USE OF UNORTHODOX TREATMENTS

The pattern of factor loadings and correlations suggests that anxiety is motivating or energizing patients into trying UTs, specifically SSUTs and faith related treatments. Or, in terms of coping theory (e.g Lazarus, 1981), use of UTs represents an instrumental coping strategy - patients are trying to avert the threat that RA represents by taking positive action.

However, the possibility that the direction of causality may be opposite to that suggested above should not be ignored. While problem focused, or instrumental, coping can undoubtedly serve a palliative function, by averting the threat, rechannelling the energy of anxiety, and by bolstering morale or hope, striving for mastery can in itself be stressful. Some people may simply prefer to relinquish control, abandoning themselves to their fate, as it were. That this is so is suggested by a study which showed that some individuals actually prefer diversion (listening to music) and random electric shocks to monitoring warnings of shock, even given the opportunity to react to the warnings and consequently avoid shocks (Averill and Rosenn, 1972). Arguably, of course, extending these findings to a real life situation, where the stakes are far greater, may be dubious. However, where there are strong indications that control may not be feasible - such as seemingly random disease variability - this approach may be the most adaptive.

It seems likely that the distress motivating prayer and use of a faith healer is occasioned by the belief that CMT is not helping very much. This is suggested by the correlation between these UTs and patients' ratings of CMT (RATEMED), and the loading of RATEMED on the 'faith factor'. As RATEMED does not load on the SSUT factor this is unlikely to be an important factor in motivating the use of this type of UT.

Depression

The loading of depression (D) on the SSUT factor indicates that the tendency to try SSUTs is negatively associated with depression - although, depression scores do not distinguish users from non-users of any one UT. As theoretically depression is associated with hopelessness, helplessness and apathy (Seligman, 1975; Seligman and Abramson, 1978) this result is sensible. The extent to which an initial depression limits the use of UTs rather than the use of unorthodox treatments serving a protective function cannot be determined by a consideration of this data; most likely both processes are in operation. Patients suffering from depression at the time of disease onset, or who are perhaps predisposed to react to threat with depression, would be less likely to try UTs because of the apathy associated with affective disorders. It is also the case that while trying a treatment the possibility that it might work, or is working, exists - i.e. it allows and encourages hope, the antithesis of depression, as many would see it.

Supporting the latter interpretation is the fact that several patients actually commented to the effect that they thought their use of UTs was perhaps as important from a psychological view point as a physical one. Also, many patients stressed the importance of 'frame of mind' in coping with arthritis, suggesting the importance, in terms of psychological as well as physical well-being, of not 'giving-up' but 'fighting'.

The data relating depression and UT use, in conjunction with the finding, reported above, that RATEMED is not associated with the use of SSUTs, supports the idea that use of SSUTS reflects a predisposition towards activity and problem solving coping. That the practice of exercise for their arthritis also loads on this factor is in line with this interpretation.

POSITIVE EFFECTS OF ILLNESS AND UNORTHODOX TREATMENT USE

GOODRATE (positive effects of illness) loads positively on the 'faith factor', indicating a positive association of these variables. Alternative interpretations for this result are discussed in Chapter 8. GOODRATE also loads in the same factor as acupuncture use and these two variables are negatively associated, although not quite significantly

($r_{pb}=-.224$, $p<0.06$)

Interestingly, both faith and use of SSUTS have something to recommend them, at least something to suggest that they may be serving a positive function - faith is positively associated with the ability to see something good in having arthritis, and use of SSUTS is associated with lower depression scores. There is nothing to indicate a positive function of acupuncture use. A possible explanation for this is that acupuncture use is associated with feelings of inequity which may hamper adjustment. The psychological significance of feelings of inequity are well documented (see for example, Eiser, 1980, for a review). People who turn to God and those who have used acupuncturists both feel CMT to have failed them to some extent, they may differ in that acupuncture users blame the medical profession for this failure while those who turn to God do not apportion blame. If one feels all that could be humanly done, is being done, one is perhaps more likely to turn to God than another practitioner, whereas, if one feels more could be done one is perhaps more likely to turn to another health professional, such as an acupuncturist. Use of an acupuncturist and indeed, feelings of inequity, may both arise from a poor doctor-patient relationship. This fits in with the interpretation of factor 2 as being concerned with the quality of the doctor-patient relationship.

PAIN LOCUS OF CONTROL AND UNORTHODOX TREATMENT USE

Internal Locus of Control

The internal locus of pain control scale (IPLC) is not associated with UT use. This result is surprising as it was predicted that UT users, particularly users of the SSUTs, would feel they had more personal control that non-users. First, it was thought an initial belief in personal control would predispose individuals to attempt to exercise it, and secondly, it was felt that the practice of self-help would help to foster feelings of personal control. In particular one might expect users of heat and massage to feel they had more control, as these are quite widely accepted as effective methods of pain control that individuals can administer themselves.

However, given the nature of the IPLC scale, which emphasises the cause of pain rather than control of pain, the lack of a simple association with UT use is not really that surprising; indeed, it would not be that surprising if it had been negatively associated with UT use. People who have expended considerable time and effort (not to mention money) in trying to get well, might be expected to disagree with statements such as 'I am directly responsible for my pain' and "peoples' pain results from their own carelessness". The lack of an association possibly reflects the ambiguity and inappropriateness of these statements.

The Powerful Others Scale

Patients who feel they are able to exercise some control over their pain by the use of UTs are perhaps more likely to have a low score on the powerful others locus of control (PPLC) subscale of the BPCQ - the items of which suggest the doctor is the sole controller of pain relief. PPLC and UT use are in fact associated (see below).

Specifically, PPLC loads on both the SSUT factor and the faith factor. It is not, however, significantly associated with any one type of UT. Taking a slightly different perspective, if one believes the doctors are 'all powerful' there is no point in trying anything else.

PPLC is not related to patients' experience of the helpfulness of CMT (r=.076, n.s.), hence, this latter variable cannot account for the association of the former and UT use.

It is perhaps rather surprising that a belief in the power of the doctor is negatively associated with the tendency to turn to God for help, as suggested by the factor solution. Possibly this result serves to confirm the suggestion made by some (e.g. Nichols 1983) that doctors are revered as 'omnipotent' and 'Godlike' by some patients.

Given the negative association of PPLC with non-practitioner UTs, the lack of an association of PPLC with acupuncture use (rpb=.102, n.s.) could be taken as weakly supporting the suggestion made earlier that some acupuncturist users may feel let down or disgruntled with conventional medicine and conventional medical practitioners. For patients who believe in the power of the medical profession but perhaps feel their doctors are not doing all they could, PPLC statements such as 'whether or not I am in pain depends of what the doctors do for me', and 'whether or not I continue to be in pain in the future depends on the skill of the doctors' are rather ambiguous. This ambiguity could account for the lack of a significant association between PPLC and acupunture use.

Chance Locus of Control Beliefs

A belief in non-contingency (operationalised here in terms of the chance scale of the BPCQ - CPLC) is supposed to predispose or rather lead to depression - this is the basic premise of Learned Helplessness Theory (Seligman, 1975). The data support this association - as already noted, depression and CPLC correlate significantly. According to Learned Helplessness Theory and the revised Learned Helplessness Theory (Abramson et al, 1978) this belief in the futility of action, brought about by the experience or perception of non-contingency, is responsible for the apathy associated with depression. Consequently, it was anticipated that CPLC would be negatively associated with UT use. This hypothesis is not supported.

While an overriding belief in chance might be supposed to lead to people giving up, it may also be the case that for some people such a belief is preceded by a search for control. If this is the case one would not necessarily predict a relationship between CPLC and the number of UTs tried, but would predict an association of CPLC and current use of unorthodox treatments. The evidence does not support this interpretation, however - CPLC is not correlated with the total number of UTs currently used (r=.007, n.s.).

The Pain Locus of Control Typology and Unorthodox Treatment Use

The fact that all three scales of the BPCQ load on no one factor suggests that the Wallston and Wallston (1982) health locus of control typology (see Chapter 2) aids little in the understanding of UT use. This was confirmed by comparing the mean number of different types of SSUTs and faith related treatments used by patients in the different categories of the typology using analysis of variance (for SSUT use, F=1.56, n.s.; for faith treatments, F=0.71, n.s.).

CONVENTIONAL MEDICAL TREATMENT AND UNORTHODOX TREATMENT USE

Use of Unorthodox Treatments and Compliance with Conventional Treatment

If one accepts that the use of UTs represents an implied criticism of CMT one would predict a negative association between compliance with CMT and UT use. Alternatively, if one sees use as a simple attempt to gain control one would predict a positive association of compliance with CMT and UT use. In particular one might predict a positive association between use of herbal remedies and compliance with medication regimes. In a factor analytic study by Pickering (1986) tranquillizer use was associated with the use of preparatory medicines, leading the author to suggest a 'pill taking type'.

In fact, none of the five measures of compliance (current drug use; incidence of refusing of dropping out of drugs in the past; incidence of refusing or dropping out of non-drug treatments; and use of day and night splints) are associated with the use of any UT, with one exception. Patients who had dropped out of at least one drugs treatment in the past tended to have tried a greater variety of methods for applying heat to help with their arthritis (rpb=.242, $p<0.04$). This result is re-emphasised by the pattern of factor loadings in factor six, which seems to distinguish users of self-administered physical treatments for pain (heat and massage) from medicine takers. Thus, it seems some patients may try to control their pain without recourse to medication.

Additionally, use of night splints (SPLINTN) loads on the faith factor in both solutions. The most likely explanation for this concerns the relationship of sex and UT use - both UT use and splint use are related to sex. As sex and UT use is the topic of a later section, discussion of this finding will be deferred.

The general lack of an association between compliance and UT use may possibly reflect the fact that, in some cases, compliance and UT use are positively associated while in others they are negatively associated. This is in line with the fact that some patients, when asked why they had tried UTs, implied they were looking for an alternative to CMT, while others implied they were simply trying to supplement CMT.

Patients' Ratings of CMT and Use of UTs

Patient rating of CMT (RATEMED) is associated with the use of an acupuncturist (rpb=-.266, $p<0.03$) and 'miscellaneous' UTs ($r=-.24$, $p<0.04$). In addition to these simple correlations RATEMED loads on the faith factor and along with acupuncture and chiropractor use in factor two.

The most obvious interpretation of these results is simply that when patients feel conventional medicine is not helping them very much they are likely to seek the guidance and help of somebody else, some other powerful other. Possibly, when patients apportion the blame for the failure of CMT on their doctors they seek an unorthodox practitioner, whereas, when they feel their treatment has not worked and nothing else will, they turn to God.

THE SOPHISTICATION HYPOTHESIS OF UNORTHODOX TREATMENT USE

Looking at the straightforward measures of association, patient 'sophistication' - in so much as socio-economic status (SES) and illness knowledge (SCORE) represent a valid and reliable gauge - is not related to UT use. However, the factor analysis indicates that faith is related to relatively high illness knowledge, while unorthodox practitioner use (at least acupuncture and chiropractic use) is associated with relatively low knowledge and low SES.

Clearly the way in which SCORE, SES, and unorthodox practitioner use are causally related cannot be determined with the present data. The results of the factor analysis might be taken as supporting the sophistication hypothesis - the idea that unsophisticated beliefs about illness predispose people to use unorthodox practitioners (see Chapter 4). However, the fact that SES and SCORE are not actually significantly correlated with either acupuncture or chiropractic use does not lend much support to the idea of such a direct link. An alternative interpretation is that poor illness knowledge and use of unorthodox practitioners both reflect an inadequate doctor-patient relationship, and patient SES, or rather the 'cultural gap' (Bochner, 1983) between doctors and patients in the lower socio-economic groups, is the cause, in part at least, of problems in the interaction. This explanation is not only intuitively appealing - patients are trying to meet their needs for professional support which are unfulfilled by the medical profession by the consultation of unorthodox practitioners - but also seems better able to account for the pattern of associations between variables.

The loading of SCORE on the faith factor might be taken as supporting the idea suggested in a previous section that users of spiritual/faith related UTs, while like unorthodox practitioner users, of the opinion that CMT is relatively unhelpful, differ in that they do not blame their doctors personally. Clearly if CMT does not work there are two main explanations possible: either it reflects professional negligence or incompetence on the part of the practitioner or it reflects the hopelessness/helplessness of the situation. People with a relatively good understanding of their condition and treatment (i.e. high illness knowledge) are probably less likely to blame their doctors for treatment failures (assuming their doctors are not negligent or incompetent) and more likely to feel satisfied that everything that can be done has been tried. Consequently, they do not seek alternative human intervention but devine intervention.

An alternative explanation for the loading of SCORE on the faith factor may be that these represent relatively sophisticated UTs. It was hypothesized (see Chapter 4) that the more contemporary, life-style oriented treatments, such as diet and stress management techniques would be favoured by the more 'sophisticated' patients. Many of the treatments subsumed under the heading of 'other/miscellaneous' UTs (ONO) can be seen to be stress management techniques (e.g. relaxation techniques, breathing exercises, yoga, meditation), and both ONO and use of diet (DNO) load on this faith factor. Furthermore, the extent to which patients feel something good has come out of their having RA (GOODRATE) also loads on this factor and this ability to reappraise a bad event positively can also be seen to represent a fairly sophisticated intrapsychic, cognitive coping strategy.

The relationship between specific beliefs about CMT and use of UTs was addressed using regression. Answers to those knowledge questions specifically concerned with the evaluation of treatment (Qs 4, 10, 17, 20, and 27) and prognosis (Qs 12, 15, and 18) were coded for optimism-pessimism (highest rank indicating the most pessimistic or negative answer, see Table 8.4) and regressed on use of SSUTs, faith treatments, and unorthodox practitioners. In the computation of UT use scales for this analysis, no account was taken of the number of a particular type of UT tried (e.g. the number of different ways heat was used); the number of different types of UT tried were simply summed. Alpha coefficients for the three scales were as follows: SSUT use, 0.2; practitioner use, 0.034; and use of faith, 0.481. Across all three analyses the only significant predictor was Q17, which obtained a significant beta weight in the regression on practitioner use (Beta=.25, $t=2.13$, $p<0.04$). This result indicates that users of unorthodox practitioners are more likely to feel deformities cannot be prevented than non-users. Given the reliability of the practitioner 'scale' little weight needs be given to this result.

DEMOGRAPHIC VARIABLES AND UNORTHODOX TREATMENT USE

Age

Age is associated with use of a faith healer (rpb=-.227, $P<0.05$) and loads on both the SSUT factor and the faith factor.

This finding of a negative association between age and use of SSUTs is consistent with the idea that as people get older they become more conservative, less innovative and more set in their ways. An alternative interpretation, that the motivation to try UTs (psychological distress) is less in older people, is not supported by the data.

The negative association between age and use of faith is perhaps a little surprising as religion generally assumes greater importance later in peoples' lives (Mitchell, 1980). One explanation is that the older population may be more orthodox and conventional in their religious beliefs and consequently less favourable to faith healers who might be considered rather 'fringy'. Age is not actually significantly associated with use of prayer (rpb=-.164, n.s.).

Sex

Sex loads on the faith and SSUT factors, indicating a fairly general tendency for men to use UTs less than women. There are of course many reasons why this might be.

Kristiansen (1984), reviewing the relevant literature, notes that men, when asked to put in order of priority a list of values, generally place health lower down the list than women, for whom it tends to be of prime importance. This, it is suggested, accounts for the finding that men engage less in preventive health behaviours (Kristiansen, 1984).

Similarly, it could be argued that if health is of relatively low value then a given health problem will represent less of a threat for men. This could explain the current findings regarding the relationship of gender and UT use, if one assumes that anxiety, proportional to the perceived threat, motivates 'illness behaviour'. This is intuitively sensible and is a premise comprising a part of both Coping Theory (e.g. Folkman et al, 1979) and the Health Belief Model (e.g. Becker and Rosenstock, 1984). Certainly, in the analysis of the present data set, anxiety is positively related to use of UTs. Evidence that men are less disturbed by their arthritis is unconvincing, however. The only measure of distress (either physical or mental) associated with sex is RATEPSY ($r_{pb}=-.242$, $p<0.04$) - men tending to rate their emotional reactions to RA as being less problematic than women. Furthermore, although men may not value health greatly, it seems likely that the things they do value, such as 'an exciting life', 'a sense of accomplishment', and 'freedom' (Kristiansen, 1984), would be seriously compromised by a potentially debilitating disease like RA.

An alternative explanation seems better able to account for the data and is consistent with the impression gained during the interviews.

In our society sexual stereotyping is a key component of socialization. Men are 'supposed' to be dynamic (certainly their value priorities reflect this), aggressive and above all strong (both mentally and physically); any admission of weakness is tantamount to failure. In this respect any chronic disease, but perhaps especially a disfiguring and disabling disease like RA, which might be seen as being a 'woman's illness', is extremely threatening to a man's self-image. One way of coping with this threat is by denial. Denial is a coping strategy particularly compatible with the male self-image, as making slight of pain and suffering is generally considered an indication of toughness and 'manliness'.

Not only is the use of UTs somewhat incompatible with a coping strategy of denial but it also implies a certain preoccupation with health which might be considered effeminate - remember 'men' do not care about health, they have higher ideals!

In line with this interpretation is the fact that more men than women said they had tried UTs to please somebody else, and the fact, already mentioned, that men rated the emotional distress occasioned by their arthritis as less of a problem than the women. Also, men are less compliant, especially in their use of splints (see Chapter 9) which can be seen to represent a very visible sign of weakness and disability.

Several pieces of anecdotal, impressionistic evidence also support this interpretation. One articulate and forthright man, during the interview, actually talked for a while about the affect of arthritis on his feelings of masculinity. He related that for years he had insisted on continuing to be a long distance lorry driver even though it was clearly a strain because of his arthritis and an alternative, supervisory position was available to him with the same firm. In retrospect he saw this seeming irrationality was a way of denying his disability and reasserting his masculinity - truck driving being a typically 'macho' occupation.

Another patient talked for some time about the start of his arthritis, stressing how he had always before been so strong and fit. Clearly, he had a very prominent image of himself as a strong 'manly' man and yet when asked about his emotional reactions to having RA, indicated that it had 'never been a problem', 'never bothered' him.

Another cue to this interpretation is provided by the fact that interviews with men were typically of shorter duration than those with women. Men tended to answer the questions in a very business-like, matter of fact way and did not talk about feelings. The section on their emotional reactions was particularly brief. The impression was that these men were uncomfortable talking about their feelings and found them unacceptable.

This explanation can also account for the finding that gender is more strongly associated with the use of UTs than CMTs.

According to Parsons' (1951) formulation of the sick role, individuals who accept or assume the sick role, in return for being excused their normal obligations to society - i.e. work and other roles and responsibilities - are obligated to comply with medical advice. Following medical directives is not considered effeminate - or to represent an effeminate preoccupation with health - but is expected and non-compliance is considered obstructive not manly. This social pressure to comply is also likely to counter, to some extent at least, the effects of denial.

SUMMARY

Factor analysis indicates three distinct, but not exclusive, patterns of unorthodox treatment use in the sample of RAs studied. Use of self supervised treatments, faith or intrapsychic treatments and unorthodox practitioners.

Among the most popular type of treatments are those patients decide upon and supervise for themselves - the over-the-counter herbal, homeopathic or dietary supplement remedies. Use of this type of treatment seems primarily to reflect a need to be doing something, for involvement in treatment.

Use of faith and intrapsychic types of unorthodox treatment (e.g. mediation, yoga, prayer etc.), on the other hand, tend to reflect a recognition and acceptance by patients that medical treatments cannot meet their needs. Patients using such treatments seem to be trying to cope with the situation rather that rectify it. Users tend to be well-informed and are likely to have a good relationship with their doctors.

The pattern of use associated with acupuncture and chiropractic use is less clearly defined in this analysis but it seems likely that it reflects a dissatisfaction with medical treatment which possibly stems from a poor doctor-patient relationship.

Notably, unorthodox treatment use, in this sample, even where it reflects dissatisfaction with conventional medical treatment, is not implicated in non-compliance with medical advice. Indeed, the majority of behaviour subsumed under the heading of unorthodox treatment use appears to be aimed at meeting needs that orthodox treatments do not, i.e. they are used to supplement orthodox treatments. Possible implications of this finding for medical practice are discussed in the following chapter.

CHAPTER 11

CONCLUSIONS

The starting point for this study was a series of very open and unstructured interviews with 18 RAs in which patients were asked about their experience of RA. It is easy to get swept along by the literature on the psychology of physical illness into asking what are, in the event, rather esoteric and irrelevant questions. These initial interviews comprised an attempt to avoid this pitfall. From these discussions a number of topics in fact emerged as being worthy of further study: patient knowledge, adjustment, compliance with medical advice and use of unorthodox treatments (UTs). The main study described in this book comprised an investigation of the predictors and interrelationship of these variables.

In terms of previous research with RAs this study is fairly distinctive. The psychological literature on RA, although quite sizeable, is dominated by investigations of the 'psychosomatic hypothesis' - the idea that psychological stress or personality variables can affect disease onset or prognosis. Research looking at patient knowledge (typically intervention studies) and compliance in RA generally has very little psychological content, as indeed, do the couple of studies which have looked at UT use in arthritics (Kronenfeld, 1982; and Elder and Acheson, 1970). Psychological distress has generally only been considered in the context of the 'psychosomatic hypothesis' or in predominantly descriptive studies.

Regarding the issue of patients' knowledge, for example, I have come across only one previous study of RAs in which the content of patients' knowledge and misconceptions was actually reported (Grennan, 1978), and this provides only a very incomplete assessment. In the present study an attempt was made to provide a much more comprehensive analysis of the content of RA patients' knowledge and misconceptions.

The results of the study support research with other patient samples with has suggested that patients actually know very little about their illness and treatment. Probably the most important finding from this component of the study, however, was that patients tended to overestimate the risks of RA and underestimate the value of their treatments - there is what was termed a 'negative bias' evident in their illness beliefs. This is interesting for a number of reasons. Practically it amplifies the need for good and systematic information to be presented to patients. The argument that patients are better off without information, that information will only worry them, really cannot be sustained in the face of this evidence.

The involved nature of some of the misconceptions patients held about their illness and treatment and their specificity to RA suggests the need for research detailing the knowledge and misconceptions of patients suffering from different illnesses. This research also suggests the need to identify an hierarchy of patient informational need. People can only take in a limited amount of information at any one time, therefore it is important that the right sort of information is highlighted at the right time. Prognostic information is likely to be important early on in all illnesses but the need for and timing of other types of information is likely to be more illness specific.

Undoubtedly the major contribution of this study to the field relates to its consideration of health behaviour and in particular UT use. Previous research on UT use is seriously limited, both in terms of quantity and quality. In the present study an attempt to consider the whole range of 'illness behaviour' undertaken by the sample studied makes it unusual. Previously researchers have tended to concentrate on compliance with conventional medical treatment or else on use of a single UT.

Factor analysis suggested the distinction of four major categories of health behaviour: compliance with conventional medical treatments; use of 'self-supervised UTs (SSUTs); use of unorthodox practitioners; and intrapsychic and faith related behaviours (e.g. prayer, use of a faith healer and re-evaluation of circumstances).

From a practical point of view the finding that compliance with conventional medical treatment is unrelated to the use of UTs is perhaps particularly important. The fact that UTs are viewed as complementary to conventional medical treatment and not as alternatives (at least in this sample) has certain implications for the medical profession concerning their attitudes to UT use. Many patients reported that their admission to their doctor that they were using an UT was received with a certain hostility. Clearly one justification for this response is refuted.

Other potential reasons for dissuading patients from UT use are also refuted by the results of this study.

While it is clear that UT use is positively associated with psychological distress, the strength of the association in no way supports the contention that their use represents psychiatric behaviour. Rather there is reason to believe their use represents a fairly successful coping strategy, motivated by psychological distress. All forms of health behaviour (including the use of conventional medical treatments) are positively associated with psychological distress, but there is some indication that use of UTs, at least 'SSUTs' and faith, promotes positive adjustment - faith related UTs are associated with the experience of positive effects of illness and use of SSUTs with lower depression scores.

The data also refute the idea that UT users are misguided by virtue of being 'unsophisticated'. The most popular UTs, SSUTs, are simply not associated with the two indices of 'sophistication' used in this study (i.e. socio-economic status and illness knowledge). While patients who turn to religious faith are actually more knowledgeable than those who do not . Only one group of UT users - users of unorthodox practitioners - are actually less 'sophisticated' than non-users and, arguably, this result is best explained in terms of the association of the quality of the doctor-patient relationship and socio-economic status demonstrated in other studies.

The extent to which this information concerning the characteristics of UT users and the relationship of use with compliance with conventional medical treatment, assuming it filters through, will change doctors' attitudes to UTs is difficult to say. Use of UTs still represents a challenge to the 'omnipotent' status which it is argued the medical profession enjoys. Certainly, the use of UTs (with the exception of unorthodox practitioners) by patients in this study was inversely associated with a 'powerful other' locus of pain control orientation, and use of both unorthodox practitioners and faith was associated with relatively low ratings of the helpfulness of conventional medical treatment.

Political and ideological reasons for using UTs, although evident, were not in high profile in this sample. However, it is my opinion that they will become increasingly important in shaping patient behaviour over the next few years.

The use of drugs as a long-term solution is becoming evermore frowned upon by the lay population - drugs are no longer considered the panacea they were once thought to be. The emphasis on way of life and more holistic treatments is becoming generally appreciated and with it the role of the medical profession more defined.

For a not unrelated reason political or consumeristic motivations for UT use are likely to become more prevalent. As it is realised that the medical profession doesn't have all the answers, their omnipotent and god-like status will be undermined and they will increasingly be seen as a commodity to 'shop around for'. In some instances UTs may be seen as viable alternatives (rather than as complementary) which they largely were not in this study.

These changes in public opinion are clearly hypothetical and research is needed to monitor changes and trends in the use of UTs. However, assuming they are evident, it is my opinion that these changes augur well for both the public and the medical profession. It seems likely that much tension and dissatisfaction on both the part of doctor and patient is caused by the patients misguided expectations of the medical profession. As the role of the doctor becomes more defined and understood by both parties these problems should diminish. Additionally, it is likely that less medical time will be taken up in consultations with patients for whom physical medicine can offer nothing - this should also increase doctor satisfaction.

Although, as I have said, such changes are likely to be seen, to some extent, over the next decade in any case, there is much to recommend their promotion.

One way of encouraging these changes is via public education. I would like to see the mutual participation style of doctor-patient interaction, as described by Szasz and Hollander (1956), promoted as I believe this will lead to the greatest patient satisfaction and service. To this end health education directed at defining doctor and patient roles and encouraging patient consumerism or assertiveness is indicated. It needs to be recognised that doctors do not have all the answers, are not infallible, differ in opinions and are susceptible to consumer pressure - basically that it is up to clients to use their doctor appropriately and intelligently.

Arguably, to successfully institute such a radical change in public opinion across all facets of society, one has to target the young. Health education sessions at secondary school represent an ideal opportunity. Certainly, I would like to see a school health education research project aimed at demystifying the medical profession and in promoting a consumer orientated or assertive patient approach. The success of the intervention could be assessed by comparing 'experimental' and control subjects during doctor-patient interviews and subsequent patient satisfaction over a given period.

Another way of promoting these changes is by targeting patient groups, especially the chronically ill such as RAs. Specifically I should like to see patient support groups institutionalized into medical practice, such that consultants recommend attendance at a course of sessions and follow-up sessions as part of the treatment regimen.

As well as providing patients with conventional counselling and information of the sort indicated in this research, one of the primary aims of such courses should be to turn patients into discerning consumers. Clearly in order to achieve this aim patients will need to be given information about available resources and facilities and how to make best use of them. For many this might also include a programme of patient assertion training in order for patients to effect the greatest use of their consultant.

In this study the majority of UT use - in particular use of SSUTs - seemed to reflect a need for activity and involvement in self-help on the part of the patients. Arguably this need is not being catered for by conventional medical treatment, although the potential to do so is there in the case of the treatment of RA. This desire for self-help could be developed in patient support sessions.

From the pilot studies it became apparent that the majority of patients were very unclear about the practice of exercise/rest, despite the fact that most had, at some time, seen a physiotherapist and were in regular contact with the occupational therapy unit. Clearly then, this is one area into which some of the patients' enthusiasm for self-help could be diverted.

Another area which might be developed concerns the use of pain management techniques. Despite the fact that RA is a particularly painful condition, few patients had received professional advice about pain management and for reasons outlined in Chapter 1 the use of analgesics is to be discouraged.

The accumulation and dissemination of information about UTs would also seem an appropriate concern for such support groups. Whether the medical profession approves of their use or not, the sheer volume of use indicates a need for patients to have access to a good source of information about UTs. For example, certain UTs can be dangerous for RAs. In particular, manipulation of the joints of the neck in RA can result in paralysis and even death. Clearly, patients need to be told about such risks. Ideally, however, patients should also be provided with more positive information about UTs, such as the names and addresses of qualified practitioners; and feedback about the benefits of use from other patients and scientific research.

The finding that male RAs are less likely to practice health behaviours than women (if substantiated) suggests a possible need to make special provision for men. The feeling that the practice of health behaviour is in some way effeminate might be countered by holding special support groups for men. Certainly, with the number of women attending the rheumatology clinic outnumbering the men four to one, there is a need to avoid a situation where men are totally overwhelmed by women.

Ideally the setting up of institutionalized support groups should be founded on research, with dependent variables including patient satisfaction and behaviour. While initially such support may seem prohibitively expensive, in terms of personnel time and uptake of services, at least for a national health service such as Britains, it seems likely that long-term economic studies would indicate a complementary reduction in terms of doctor-patient consultation time. It seems very likely that the professional support patients at present get (in this sample, typically two ten minute visits to the consultant per year) leads to a great number of irrelevant and unsuccessful visits to busy G.P.s.

Certainly, I feel the proportion of medical staff to support and paramedical staff needs rebalancing. Doctors are relatively highly paid (even in Britain) specialists and they should be used as such. This does not mean they should be unapproachable, but emotional support and patient educational needs (which at the present consume a great proportion of medical time) could be provided for more economically and probably more effectively and sensitively elsewhere. Patient need is unlikely to diminish and, therefore, until alternative care provision is made and promoted it is likely that doctors will continue to be used inappropriately.

REFERENCES

Aakster, C.W. (1986) Concepts in alternative medicine. Social Science in Medicine, 22, 265-273.

Abramson, L.Y. and Seligman , M.E.P. (1978) Learned helplessness in humans: Critique and reformulation. Journal of Abnormal Psychology, 87, 49-74.

Achterberg, J., McGraw, P., and Lawlis, G.F. (1981). Rheumatoid arthritis: A study of relaxation and temperature biofeedback training as an adjunctive therapy. Biofeedback and Self-Regulation, 6, 207-223.

Achterberg-Lawlis, J. (1982). The psychological dimensions of arthritis. Journal of Consulting and Clinical Psychology, 50, 984-992.

Adler, R. (Ed.). (1981). Psychoneuroimmunology. New York: Academic Press.

Aitken-Swan, J. and Easson, E.C. (1959). Reactions of cancer patients on being told their diagnosis. British Medical Journal, 1, 779-781.

Alexander, F. (1950). Psychosomatic Medicine. New York: Norton.

American Rheumatism Association (1959). Diagnostic criteria for rheumatoid arthritis, 1958 revision. Annals of the Rheumatic Diseases, 18, 49-53.

Amkraut, A., Soloman, G.F., and Kraemer, H.C. (1971). Stress, early experience and adjuvant-induced arthritis in the rat. Psychosomatic Medicine, 33, 203-214.

Anderson, C.D., Stoyva, J.M., and Vaughn, L.J. (1982). A test of delayed recovery following stressful stimulation in four psychosomatic disorders. Journal of Psychosomatic Research, 26, 571-580.

Anderson, K.O., Bradley, L.A., Young, L.D., and McDaniel, L.K. (1985). Rheumatoid arthritis: Review of psychological factors related to etiology, effects, and treatment. Psychological Bulletin, 98(2), 358-387.

Arthritis and Rheumatism Council (1985). Rheumatoid Arthritis Explained: A Handbook for Patients.

Atkinson, J.W. (1957). Motivational determinants of risk-taking behaviour. Psychological Review, 64, 359-372.

Averill, J.R. and Rosenn, M. (1972). Vigilant and non-vigilant coping stategies and psychophysiological stress reactions during the anticipation of electric shock. Journal of Personality and Social Psychology, 23 128-141.

Avina, R.L. and Schneider, L.J. (1978). Why patients choose homeopathy. Western Journal of Medicine, 128, 366-369. Ballantine, H.T. (1972). Will the delivery of health care be improved by the use of chiropractic services? New England Journal of Medicine, 286 237.

Barquero, V.J.L. (1982). The General Health Questionnaire as an instrument for screening psychiatric pathology in cardiac patients. (Abstract) Actas Luso-Espanolas de Neurologia y Psiqriatria y Gencias Afines, 10, 21-32.

Barratt, P.T. and Kline, P. (1981). The observation to variable ratio in factor analysis. Personality Study and Group Behaviour, 1, 23-33.

Bartrop, R.W., Luckhurst, E., Lazarus, L., Kiloh, L.G., and Penny, R. (1977). Depressed lymphoyte function after bereavement. Lancet, 1, 834-836.

Beard, B.H. (1969). Fear of death and fear of life: The dilemma in chronic renal failure, heamodialysis, and kidney transplantation. Archives of General Psychiatry, 21, 373-380.

Beck, A.T. (1978). Depression Inventory. Philadelphia Centre for Cognitive Therapy.

Becker, M.H. (1976). Sociobehavioural determinants of compliance. In D.L. Sackett and R.B. Haynes (Eds.), Compliance with Therapeutic Regimens. Baltimore: Johns Hopkins University Press.

Becker, M.H., Drachman, R.H., and Kirsch, J.P. (1972). Predicting mother's compliance with pediatric medical regimens. Journal of Pediatrics, 81, 843-854.

Becker, M.H. and Maiman, L.A. (1975). Sociobehavioural determinants of compliance with health and medical care recommendations. Medical Care, 13, 10-24.

Becker, M.H., Radius, S.M., Rosenstock, I.M., Drachman, R.H., Schubert, K.C., and Teets, K.C. (1978). Compliance with a medical regimen for asthma: A test of the health belief model. Public Health Report, 93, 268-277.

Becker, M.H. and Rosenstock, I.M. (1984). Compliance with medical advice. in A. Steptoe and A. Mathews (Eds.), Health Care and Human Behaviour. London: Academic Press.

Beisser, A.R. (1979). Denial and affirmation in illness and health. American Journal of Psychiatry , 136, 1026-1030.

Belcon, M.C., Haynes, R.B., and Tugwell, P. (1984). A critical review of compliance studies in rheumatoid arthritis. Arthritis and Rheumatism, 27, 1227-1233.

Ben-Sira, Z. (1981). The structure of readjustment of the disabled: An additional perspective on rehabilitation. Social Science and Medicine, 15A, 565-580.

Ben-Sira, Z. (1982). Lay evaluation of medical treatment and competence: Development of a model of the function of the physician's affective behaviour. Social Science and Medicine, 16, 1013-1019.

Ben-Sira, Z. (1983). Loss stress and readjustment: The structure of coping with bereavement and disability. Social Science and Medicine, 17, 1619-1632.

Bender, M.O. (1965). Pathway to Chiropractic Utilization: A Preliminary Study. Columbia University, School of Public Health and Administrative Medicine: unpublished report.

Berger, M., Bobbitt, R.A., Carter, W.B., and Gilson, B.S. (1981). The sickness impact profile: Development and trial revision of a health status measure. Medical Care, 19, 787-805.

Berkman, L. and Syme, S.L. (1979). Social networks, host resistance, and mortality: A nine year follow-up study of Alameda County residents. American Journal of Epidemiology, 100(2), 186-204.

Berkowitz, N.H., Malone, M.F., and Klein, M.W., (1963). Patient follow-through in the outpatient department. Nursing Research, 12, 16-22.

Bertakis, K.D. (1977). The communication of information from the physician to patient: A method for increasing retention and satisfaction. Journal of Family Practice, 5, 217-222.

Bhatt-Sanders, D. (1985). Acupuncture for rheumatoid arthritis: An analysis of the literature. Seminars in Artritis and Rheumatism, 14, 225-231.

Blackburn, J.C. and Hindmarsh, K.W. (1976). Corticosteroids contained in Mexican cures for arthritis and asthma. Canadian Medical Association Journal, 114, 299-302.

Blom, G.E., and Nicholls, G. (1954). Emotional factors in children with rheumatoid arthritis. American Journal of Orthopsychiatry, 24, 588-601.

Bochner, S. (1983). Doctors, patients and their cultures. In D. Pendleton and J. Hasler (Eds.), Doctor-Patient Communication. London: Academic Press.

Booth, G.C. (1937). Personality and chronic arthritis. Journal of Nervous Mental Disease, 85, 637-645.

Bowestom, N.C. and Howard, M.T. (1965). Personality characteristics of three disability groups. Archives of Physical Medicine and Rehabilitation, 46, 626-632.

Bowlby, J. (1960). Grief and mourning in infancy and early childhood. Psychoanalytic Study of the Child, 15, 9-52.

Bowlby, J. (1961). Processes of mourning. The International Journal of Psychoanalysis, 42, 317-340.

Boyd, T.R., Covington, T.R., Stanaszek, W.F., and Coussons, R.T. (1974). Drug defaulting. Part 4: Analysis of non-compliance patterns. American Journal of Hospital Pharmacy, 31, 485-491.

Bradshaw, P.W., Ley, P., Kincey, J.A., and Bradshaw, J. (1975). Recall of medical advice comprehensibility and specificity. British Journal of Social and Clinical Psychology, 14, 55-62.

Bray, G. P. (1978). Rehabilitation of spinal cord injured: A family approach. Journal of Applied Rehabilitation Counselling, 9, 70-78.

Breen, A.C. (1977). Chiropractors and the treatment of back pain. Rheumatology and Rehabilitation, 16, 46.

British Medical Association (1986). Alternative Therapy: Report.

Brody, D.S. (1980). An analysis of patient recall of their therapeutic regimens. Journal of Chronic Diseases, 33, 57-63.

Brooks, P.M. and Lowenthal, R.M. (1977). Chinese herbal arthritis cures in agranulocytosis. Medical Journal of Australia, 2, 860-861.

Brown, J.H., Kazis, L.E., Spitz, P.W., Gertman, P., Fries, J.F., and Meenan, R.F. (1984). The dimensions of health outcomes: A cross-validated examination of health status measurement. American Journal of Public Health, 74, 159-161.

Brown, J.S., Perman, B.S., and Dobbs, J.L. (1981). The will to live. Research of Aging, 3, 182-201.

Brown, G.W., Davidson, S., Harris, T., Maclean, U., Pollack, S., and Prudo, S. (1977). Psychiatric disorder in London and North Uist. Social Science and Medicine, 11, 367-77.

Brown, G.W. and Harris, T. (1978). Social Origins of Depression: A study of Psychiatric Disorder in Women. Tavistock Publications.

Bruhn, J.G., Hampton, J.W., and Chandler, B.C. (1971). Clinical marginality and psychological adjustment in haemophilia. Journal of Psychosomatic Research, 15, 207-213.

Burt, C. and Banks, C. (1947). A factor analysis of body measurements for British adult males. Annal of Eugenics, 13, 238-256.

Butler, J. (1980). The Utilization of Alternative Health Services. Unpublished Doctoral Dissertation: George Peabody College for Teachers of Vanderbuilt University. Butt, H.R. (1977). A method for better physician-patient communication. Annals of Internal Medicine, 86, 478-480.

Byrne, P.S. and Long, B.E. (1976). Doctors Talking to Patients. London: Her Majesty's Stationary Office.

Carpenter, J.O. and Davis, L.J. (1976). Medical recommendations - followed or ignored. Archives of Physical and Medical Rehabilitation, 57, 241-245.

Casel, E.J. (1976). Disease as an it: Concepts of disease as revealed by patients' presentation of symptons. Social Science Medicine, 10, 143-146.

Cassileth, B.R., Lusk, E.J., Strouse, T.B., and Bodenheimer, B.J. (1984). Contempory unorthodox treatments in cancer medicine: A study of patients, treatments and practitioners. Annals of Internal Medicine, 101, 105-112.

Cattell, R.B. (1965). The Scientific Analysis of Personality. Chicago: Aldine Publishing Co.

Cattell, R.B. (1966). The Scree Test for the number of factors. Multivariate Behavioural Research, 1, 245-276.

Cattell, R.B. (1978). The Scientific Use of Factor Analysis in Behavioural and Life Sciences. New York: Plenum Press.

Christie, M.J. (1975). The psychosocial environment and precursors of disease. In P.H. Venables and M.J. Christie (Eds.), Research in Psychophysiology. New York: Wiley.

Classifications of Occupations and Coding Index. (1980) H.M.S.O., O.F.P.C.S

Cleary, P.D. (1982). Chiropractic use: A test of several hypotheses. American Journal of Public Health, 72, 727.

Cleveland, S.E. and Fisher, S. (1960). A comparison of psychological characteristics and physiological reactivity in ulcer and rheumatoid arthritis groups: I. Psychological measures. Psychosomatic Medicine, 22, 283-289.

Cleveland, S.E., Reitman, E.E., and Brewer, E.J., Jr. (1965). Psychological factors in juvenile rheumatoid arthritis. Arthritis and Rheumatism, 8, 1152-1157.

Clum, G., Scott, L., and Burnside, J.(1979). Information and locus of control as factors in the outcomes of surgery. Psychological Reports, 45, 867-873.

Cobb, S. (1976). Social support as a moderator of life stress. Psychosomatic Medicine, 38, 300-314.

Cobb, S., Bauer, W., and Whiting, I. (1939). Environmental factors in rheumatoid arthritis: A study of the relation between onset and exacerbation of rheumatoid arthritis and emotional or environmental factors. Journal of the American Medical Association, 111, 668-670.

Cobb, S., Kasl, S.V, Chen, E., and Christenfeld, R., (1965). Some psychological and social characteristics of patients hospitalized for rheumatoid arthritis, hypertension, and duodenal ulcer. Journal of Chronic Diseases, 18, 1259-1278.

Cobb, S., Miller, M., and Wieland, M. (1959). On the relationship between divorce and rheumatoid arthritis. Arthritis and Rheumatism, 2, 214-218.

Cochrane, R. and Sobel, M. (1980). Life stress and psychological consequences. In P. Feldman and J. Orford (Eds.), Psychological Problems: The Social Contract. Wiley.

Coe, R.M. (1978). Sociology of Medicine. Second edition. New York: McGraw-Hill.

Cohn, N.K. (1961). Understanding the process of adjustment to disability. Journal of Rehabilitation, 27, 16-18.

Consumer Report (1979). The mistreatment of arthritis. Consumer Report, June, 340-343.

Cooper, S.E. (1983). Some social-demographic characteristics of patients self referred for a clinical trial of laetril. Journal of Psychosocial Oncology, 1, 83-91.

Cormier, B.M., Wittkower, E.D., Marcotte, V., and Forget, F. (1957). Psychological aspects of rheumatoid arthritis. Canadian Medical Association Journal, 77, 533.

Coulehan, F.L. (1985). Chiropractic and the clinical art. Social Science and Medicine, 21, 383-390.

Counti, M.A., Pavlon, M., and Hartings, M. (1978). The use of non-medical treatments (chiropractics, acupuncture, miracle diets, psychic surgery) by multiple sclerosis patients. Sociological Symposium, 22, 55-74.

Coyne, J.C. and Lazarus, R.S. (1980). Cognitive style, stress perception, and coping. In I.L. Kutash and L.B. Schlesinger (Eds.), Handbook on Stress and Anxiety: Contemporary Knowledge Theory and Treatment. San Francisco: Jossey-Bass.

Cromwell, R.L. and Levenkron, J.C. (1984). Psychological care of acute coronary patients. In A. Steptoe and A. Mathews (Eds.), Health Care and Human Behaviour. London Academic Press.

Cronbach, L.J. (1951). Coefficient alpha and the internal structure of tests. Psychometrika, 16, 297-334.

Crown, S. and Crisp, A.H. (1966). A short clinical diagnostic self-rating scale for psychoneurotic patients. The Middlesex Hospital Questionnaire (M.H.Q.). British Journal of Psychiatry, 112 917-923.

Crown, S. and Crown, J.M. (1973). Personality in early rheumatoid disease. Journal of Psychosomatic Research, 17, 189-196.

Crown, S., Crown, J.M., and Fleming, A. (1975). Aspects of the psychology and epidemiology of rheumatoid disease. Psychological Medicine, 5, 291-299.

Cushing, H. (1925). The Life of Sir William Osler, Vol I. New York: Oxford University Press.

Davidson, T.N., Bowden, M.L., and Feller, I. (1981). Social support and post-burn adjustment. Archives of Physical Medicine and Rehabilitation, 62, 274-278.

DeCastro, F.J. (1972). Doctor-patient communication. Clinical Pediatrics, 11, 86-87.

Denver, D.R., Laveault, D., Girard, F., Lacourciere, Y., Latulippe, L., Grove, R.N., Preve, M., and Doiron, N. (1979). Behavioural medicine: Biobehavioural effects of short-term thermal biofeedback and relaxation in rheumatoid arthritis patients (abstract). Biofeedback and Self-Regulation, 4, 245-246.

DeVellis, R.F., DeVellis, B.M., Wallston, B.S., and Wallston, K.A. (1980). Epilepsy and learned helplessness. Basic and Applied Social Psychology, 1, 241-253.

DeVon, H.A. and Powers. M.J. (1984). Health beliefs, adjustment to illness and control of hypertension. Research in Nursing and Health, 7, 10-16.

DeWet, B. and Hollingshead, J. (1980). Medicine compliance in paediatric out-patients. South African Medical Journal, 58, 846-848.

D.H.S.S. (1980). Inequalities in Health: A Report of a Research Working Group. London: D.H.S.S.

Dlin, B.M., Fischer, J.L., and Huddell, B. (1968). Psychologic adaptation to pacemaker and open-heart surgery. Archives of General Psychiatry, 19, 599-610.

Dohrenwend, B.P. and Dohrenwend, B.S. (1974). Psychiatric disorders in urban settings. In G. Caplan (Ed.), American Handbook of Psychiatry,Vol II: Child and Adolescent Psychiatry, Sociocultural and Community Psychiatry. New York: Basic Books.

Dollard, J. and Miller, N.E. (1950). Personility and Psychotherapy. McGraw-Hill.

Donham, G.W., Ladenig, K., Snads, M.M., and Holzer, P.D. (1983). Personality correlates of health locus of control with medical in-patients. Journal of Psychological Reports, 52, 659-666.

Dove, C.I (1976). Alternative medicine: Osteopathy. Nursing Times, 72, 129-31.

Downie, W.W., Leatham, P.A., Rhind, V.M., Wright, V., Brancho, J.A., and Anderson, J.A. (1978). Studies with pain rating scales. Annal of Rheumatic Diseases, 37, 378-381.

Dubuisson, D. and Melzack, R. (1976). Classification of clinical pain descriptions by multiple group discriminant analysis. Experimental Neurology , 51, 480-487.

Duff, R. and Hollinghead, A. (1968). Sickness and Society. New York: Harper and Row.

Duthie, J.J.R. (1957). Textbook of the Rheumatic Diseases. Edinburgh: Churchill Livingstone.

Duthie, J.J.R., Brown, P.E., Truelove, L.H., Baragar, F.D., and Lawrie, A.J. (1964). Course and prognosis in rheumatoid arthritis: A final report. Annals of Rheumatic diseases, 23, 193-202.

Earle, J.R., Perricone, P.J., Maultsby, D.M., Perricone, N., Turner, R.A., and Davis, J. (1979). Psychosocial adjustment of rheumatoid arthritis patients from two alternative treatment settings. Journal of Rheumatology, 6, 80-87.

Edwards, H. (1975). Alternative medicine: the science of spiritual healing. Nursing Times, 71, 2008-2010.

Edwards, W., (1974). The theory of decision making. Psychological Bulletin, 51, 380-417.

Ehrlich, G.E. (1982). Diagnosis and management of rheumatic diseases in older patients. Journal of the American Geriatrics Society, 30, 45-51.

Eiser, J.R. (1980). Cognitive Social Psychology: A Guide to Theory and Research. Maidenhead: McGraw-Hill.

Ekland, L.H. and Wessling, A. (1976). Evaluation of package enclosures for drug packages. Lakaridningen, 73, 2319-2310.

Elder, R. and Acheson, R.M. (1970). New Haven survey of joint disease XIV. Social class and behaviour in response to symptoms of osteoarthritis. Millbank Memorial Fund Quarterly, 48, 448-501.

Ell, K.O. (1985-86). Coping with serious illness: On integrating constructs to enhance clinical research, assessment and intervention. International Journal of Psychiatry in Medicine, 15, 335-356.

Ellis, D.A., Hopkins, J., Letch, A.G., and Crofton, S. (1979). Doctors' orders: Controlled trial of supplementary written information for patients. British Medical Journal, 1 456.

Engel, B.T. (1972). Response specificity . In N.S. Greenfield and R.A. Sternbach (Eds.), Psychophysiological Handbook. New York: Holt,Rinehart and Winston.

Engel, G.L. (1962). Psychological Development in Health and Disease. Philadelphia: Saunders.

Engel, G.L. (1964). Grief and grieving. American Journal of Nursing, 64, 93-98.

Evans, R.L. and Northwood, L.R. (1983). Social support needs in adjustment to stroke. Archives of Physical Medicine and Rehabilitation, 64, 61-63.

Eysenck, H.J. and Eysenck, S.B.G. (1964). Manual of the Eysenck Personality Inventory. University of London Press: London.

Fabrega, H. and Silver, D. (1973). Illness and Shamanistic Caring in Zinacanton. Stanford University Press: Stanford, CA.

Feinstein, A., Wood, H.F., Epstein, J.A., Taranta, A., Simpson, R., and Tursky, E. (1959). A controlled study of three methods of prophylaxis against streptococcal infection in a population of rheumatic children:II. Results of the first three years of the study, including methods for evaluating the maintenance of oral prophylaxis. New England Journal of Medicine, 260, 697-702.

Felton, B.T. and Revenson, T.A. (1984). Coping with chronic illness: A study of illness controllability and influence of coping strategies on psychological adjustment. Journal of Consulting and Clinical Psychology, 52, 343-53.

Ferguson, K. and Boyle, G.G. (1979). Family support, health beliefs, and therapeutic compliance in patients with rheumatoid arthritis. Patient Counselling and Health Education, 1, 101-105.

Festinger, L. (1957). A Theory of Cognitive Dissonance. Evanston, III: Row, Peterson.

Firman, G.J. and Goldstein, M.S. (1975). The future of chiropractic: A psychosocial view. New England Journal of Medicine, 293, 639.

Fishbein, M. and Ajzen, I. (1975). Beliefs, Attitude, Intention, and Behaviour: An Introduction to Theory and Research. Reading, Mass: Addison-Wesley.

Fisher, E. (1971). Patients' evaluation of out-patient medical care. Journal of Medical Education, 46, 238-48.

Fisher, S. and Cleveland, S. (1960). A comparison of psychological characteristics and physiological reactivity in ulcer and rheumatoid arthritis groups. Psychosomatic Medicine, 22, 290-293.

Fitzgerald, R.C. (1970). Reactions to blindness: An exploratory study of adults with recent loss of sight. Archives of General Psychiatry, 22, 370-379.

Folkman, S. and Lazarus, R.S. (1980). An analysis of coping in a middle-aged community sample. Journal of Health and Social Behaviour, 21, 219-239.

Folkman, S., Schaefer, C., and Lazarus, R.S. (1979). Cognitive processes as mediators of stress and coping. In V. Hamilton and D.M. Warburton (Eds.), Human Stress and Cognition: An Information-Processing Approach. John Wiley and Sons.

Francis, W., Korsch, B.M., and Morris, M.J. (1969). Gaps in doctor-patient communication: Patients' response to medical advice. New England Journal of Medicine, 280, 535-540.

Freer, C.B. (1985). What kind of alternative is alternative medicine? Journal of the Royal College of General Practitioners, 35 (279), 459-460.

French, C., Mellor, M., and Parry, L. (1978). Patients' views of the ophthalmic optician. Ophthalmic Optician, 28 October, 784-786.

Freyberger, H. (1980). Renal transplant unit. Advances in Psychosomatic Medicine, 10, 151-177.

Fries, J.F., Spitz, P., Kraines, R.G., and Holman, H.R. (1980). Measurement of patient outcome in arthritis. Arthritis and Rheumatism, 23, 137-145.

Fries, J.F., Spitz, P.W., and Young, P.Y. (1982). The dimensions of health outcomes: The Health Assessment Questionnaire, Disability and Pain Scales. Journal of Rheumatology, 9, 789-793.

Gardiner, B.M. (1980). Psychological aspects of rheumatoid arthritis. Psychological Medicine, 10, 159-163.

Geersten, H.R., Gray, R.M., and Ward, J.R. (1973). Patient non-compliance within the context of seeking medical care for arthritics. Journal of Chronic Diseases, 26, 689-698.

Gerle, B., Lundon, G., and Sandblom, P. (1960). The patient with inoperable cancer from the psychiatric and social standpoints. Cancer, 13, 1206-1211.

Gibson, R.G., Gibson, S.L.M., MacNeill, A.D., and Buchanan, W.W. (1980). Homeopathic therapy in rheumatoid arthritis: Evaluation by double blind clinical therapeutic trial. British Journal of Clinical Pharmacy, 9, 453-459.

Gilbertsen, V.A. and Wangensteen, O.H. (1962). Should the doctor tell the patient that the disease is cancer? Ca: A Cancer Journal for Clinicians, 12, 82-86.

Goldberg, D. (1967). The Assessment of the Severity of Non-Psychotic Psychiatric Illness by Means of a Questionnaire. Unpublished D.P.M. Dissertation: University of London.

Goldberg, D. (1972). The Detection of Psychiatric Illness by Questionnaire. Maudsley Monograph No. 21, O.U.P.

Goldberg, D. (1978). Manual of the General Health Questionnaire. Windsor,Berks: NFER Publishing Co.

Goldberg, D., Cooper, D., Eastwood, M., Kedward, H., and Sheperd, M. (1970). A psychiatric interview suitable for use in community surveys. British Journal of Preventative Medicine, 24, 18-26.

Goldberg, D.P. and Hillier, V.F. (1979). A scaled version of the General Health Questionnaire. Psychological Medicine, 9, 139-145.

Goldberg, D. and Huxley, P. (1980). Mental Illness in the Community: The Pathway to Psychiatric Care. London and New York: Tavistock Publications.

Goldberg, E.M. and Morrison, S.L. (1963). Schizophrenia and social class. British Journal of Psychiatry, 109, 785-802.

Goldberg, I., Babigian, H.M., Locke, B., and Rosen, B. (1974). Role of non-psychiatrist physicians in the delivery of mental health services: Implications from three studies. Public Health Reports, 93, 240-45.

Goldstein, L. (1980). Relationship of Health Locus of Control and Individual Diabetic Management. Unpublished Masters' Thesis: Pace University.

Gordis, L., Markowitz, M., and Lilienfeld, A. (1969). The inaccuracy of using interviews to estimate patient reliability in taking medications at home. Medical Care, 7, 49-54.

Graham, C., Bond, S.S., Gerkousch, M.M., and Cook, M.R. (1980). Use of the McGill Pain Questionnaire in the assessment of cancer pain: Replicability and consistency. Pain, 8, 377-387.

Grennan, D.M., Taylor, S., Palmer, D.G. (1978). Doctor-patient communication in patients with arthritis. New Zealand Medical Journal, 87, 431-434.

Gross, M. and Brandt, K. (1981). Educational support groups for patients with ankylosing spondylitus: A preliminary report. Patient Counselling and Health Education, 3, 6-12.

Guilford, J.P. (1953). The correlation of an item with a composite measure of the remaining items in a test. Educational and Psychological Measurement, 13, 87-93.

Gunther, M.S. (1969). Emotional aspects. In D. Reige (Ed.), Spinal Cord Injuries. Springfield, Mass: Charles C. Thomas.

Guttman, L. (1976). Spinal Cord Injuries: Comprehensive Management and Research (second edition). Oxford: Blackwell Scientific Publications.

Halliday, J.L. (1942). Psychological aspects of rheumatoid arthritis. Proceedings of the Royal Society of Medicine, 35, 455-457.

Hamilton, V. (1975). Socialization anxiety and information processing: A capacity model of anxiety-induced performance deficits. In I.G. Sarason and C.D. Spielberger (Eds.), Stress and Anxiety, Vol.II. Washington, D.C.: Hemisphere.

Hasling, M. (1975). Alternative medicine: Homeopathy. Nursing Times, 71, 1240-1242.

Harris, D.M. and Guten, S. (1979). Health-protective behaviour: An exploratory study. Journal of Health and Social Behaviour, 20, 17-29.

Hart, W.R. (1979). Rheumatoid arthritis, depression and preceding life events: A study of event desirability, anticipation, control and coping effectiveness. Dissertation Abstracts, 39 (11-13), 5556-5557.

Hathaway, S.R. and McKinley, J.C. (1967). Minnesota Multiphasic Personality Inventory Manual. New York: The Psychological Corporation.

Hatz, P.S. (1978). The Relationship of Life Satisfaction and Locus of Control in Patients Undergoing Chronic Hemodialysis. Unpublished Master's Thesis: University of Illinois.

Hauser, S.T. (1981). Physician-patient relationships. In E.G. Mishler, Social Contexts of Health, Illness and Patient Care. Cambridge University Press.

Haynes, R.B. (1976). A critical review of the "determinants" of patient compliance with therapeutic regimens. In D.L. Sackett and R.B. Haynes (Eds.), Compliance with Therapeutic Regimens. Baltimore: John Hopkins University Press.

Haynes, R.B. and Sackett, D.L. (1977). MacMaster University Compliance Bibliography . Mimeo.

Haynes, R.B., Taylor, D.W., and Sackett, D.L. (Eds.) (1979). Compliance in Health Care. Baltimore: John Hopkins University Press.

Helman, C.G. (1978). "Feed a cold, starve a fever"- Folk models of infection in an English surburban community, and their relation to medical treatment. Cultural, Medicine and Psychiatry, 2, 107-137.

Henderson, S., Duncan-Jones, P. McAuley, M., and Ritchie, K. (1978). The patients' primary group. British Journal of Psychiatry. 132, 74-86.

Hendrie, H.C., Paraskevas, F., Baragar, F.D., and Adamson, J.D. (1971). Stress, immunoglobulin levels and early polyarthritis. Journal of Psychosomatic Research, 15, 337-343.

Hermann, F. (1973). The out-patient prescription label as a source of medication errors. Americian Journal of Hospital Pharmacy, 30, 155-159.

Hermann, F., Herxheimen, A., and Lionel, N.D.W. (1978). Package inserts for prescribed medicines: What minimum information do patients need? British Medical Journal, 2, 1132-1135.

Hewer, W. (1983). The relationship between the alternative practitioner and his patient: A review. Psychotherapy and Psychosomatics, 40, 172-180.

Hiroto, D.S, (1974). Locus of control and learned helplessness. Journal of Experimental Psychology, 102, 187-193.

Hiroto, D.S. and Seligmen, M.E.P. (1975). Generality of learned helplessness in man. Journal of Personality and Social Psychology, 31, 311-327.

Hohmann, G.W. (1975). Psychological aspects of treatment and rehabilitation of the spinal cord injured person. Clinical Orthopaedics and Related Research, 112, 81-88.

House, J.S. (1981). Work Stress and Social Support. Reading, M.A: Addison-Wesley.

Hulka, B.S., Kupper, L.L., Cassel, J.C., and Efird, R.L. (1975). Medication use and misuse: Physician-patient discrepancies. Journal of Chronic Diseases, 38, 7-21.

Hunter, M., Philips, C., and Rachman, S. (1979). Memory for pain. Pain, 6, 35-46.

Huskisson, E.C. (1976). Chronopharmacology of anti-rheumatic drugs with special reference to indomethacin. In E.C. Huskisson and G.P. Velo (Eds.), Inflammatory Arthropathies. Excerpta Medica: Amsterdam.

Huskisson, E.C. and Hart, F.D. (1978). Joint Disease: All the Arthropathies. Bristol: John Wright and Son Ltd.

Huskisson, E.C., Dieppe, P.A., Tucker, A.K., and Cannell, L.B. (1979). Another look at osteoarthritis. Annals of the Rheumatic Diseases, 38, 423-428.

Huskisson, E.C., Jaffe, I.A., Scott, J., and Dieppe, P.A. (1980). 5-thiopyridoxine in rheumatoid arthritis: Clinical and experimental studies. Arthritis and Rheumatism, 23, 106-110.

Huskisson, E.C. (1983). Visual analogue scales. In R. Melzack (Ed.), Pain Measurement and Assessment. New York: Raven Press.

Janis, I. (1958). Psychological Stress: Psychoanalytic and Behavioural Studies of Surgical Patients. New York: Wiley.

Jenny, J. (1983). A compliance model for diabetic instruction. Rehabilitation Literature, 44, 258-263.

Johnstone, A. and Goldberg, D. (1976). Psychiatric screening in general practice. Lancet, 1, 605-608.

Johnson, J.E., Rice, V.H., Fuller, S.S., and Endress, M.P. (1978). Sensory information, instruction in coping strategy, and recovery from surgery. Research and Nursing Health, 1, 4-17.

Jolley, C., Feld, B., Caraway, A., Prystowsky, H. (1971). Research in the delivery of female health care: Recipients' reaction. American Journal of Obstetrics and Gynecology, 110, 291-300.

Joyce, C.R. (1962). Patient co-operation and the sensitivity of clinical trials. Journal of Chronic Diseases, 13, 1025-1076.

Kaplan, S. and Kozin, F. (1981). A controlled study of group counselling in rheumatoid arthritis. Journal of Rheumatology, 8, 91-99.

Kasl, S.V. (1974). The health belief model and behaviour related to chronic illness. Health Education Monographs, 2, 433-454.

Kasl, S.V. and Cobb, S. (1966). Health behaviour, illness behaviour, and sick role behaviour. Archives of Environmental Health, 12, 246-266 and 531-541.

Kasl, S.V. and Cobb, S. (1969). The intrafamilial transmission of rheumatoid arthritis: V. Journal of Chronic Diseases, 22, 239-258.

Kastler, J., Kane, R.L., and Olsen, D.M. (1976). Issues underlying prevalance of "doctor-shopping" behaviour. Journal of Health and Social Behaviour, 17, 328-339.

Kaye, R.L and Hammond, A.H. (1978). Understanding rheumatoid arthritis: Evaluation of a patient education program. Journal of the American Medical Association, 239, 2466-2467.

Kelly, W.D. and Friesen, S.R. (1950). Do cancer patients want to be told? Surgery, 27, 822-826.

Kelner, M., Hall, O., and Coulter, I. (1980). Chiropractors, Do They Help? Toronto: Fitzhenry and Whiteside.

Kendall, P.L. and Wolf, K.M. (1949). The analysis of deviant cases in communication research. In P.F. Lazarsfeld and F.M. Stanton (Eds.), Communications Research. New York: Harper and Brothers.

Key, M.K. (1975). Psychosocial and Education Factors Surrounding Compliance Behaviour of Hypertensives. Unpublished Doctoral Disseration: George Peabody College for Teachers.

Kiecolt-Glaser, J.K., Garner, W., Speicher, C., Penn, G.M., Holliday, J., and Glaser, R. (1984). Psychosocial modifiers of immunocompetence in medical students. Psychosomatic Medicine, 46, 7-14.

Kincey, J.A., Bradshaw, P.W., and Ley, P. (1975). patients' satisfaction and reported acceptance of advice in general practice. Journal of the Royal College of General Practitioners, 25, 558-566.

King, S.H. and Cobb, S. (1958). Psychosocial factors in the epidemiology of rheumatoid arthritis. Journal of Chronic Diseases, 7, 466-475.

Kirsch, J.P. and Rosenstock, I.M. (1979). Patients' problems in following recommendations of health experts. In G. Stone, F. Cohen, and N.E. Adler (Eds.), Health Psychology. San Francisco: Jossey-Bass.

Klein, D.C. and Seligman, M.E.P. (1976). Reversal of performance deficits in learned helplessness and depression. Journal of Abnormal Psychology, 85, 11-26.

Klinger, E. (1975). Consequences of commitment to and disengagement from incentives. Psychological Review, 82, 1-25.

Knudson, K.G., Spiegel, T.M., and Furst, D.E. (1981). Out-patient educational program for rheumatoid arthritis patients. Patient Counselling and Health Education, 3, 77-82.

Koos, E.L. (1967). The Health of Regionville. New York: Hafner Publishing Co.

Korsch, B., Freemon, B., and Negrete, V. (1971). Practical implications of doctor-patient interactions: Analysis for pediatric practice. American Journal of Diseases of Children, 121, 110-114.

Korsch, B.M., and Negrete, V.F. (1972). Doctor-patient communication. Scientific American, 227, 66-74.

Kremer, J.M., Bigauoette, J., Michalek, A.V., Timchalk, M.A., Lininger, L., Rynes, R.I., Huyck, C., Ziemiuski, J., and Bartholomew, L.E. (1985). Effects of manipulation of dietary fatty acids on clinical manifestations of rheumatoid arthritis. Lancet, 1, 184-187.

Krieger, D. (1976). Alternative medicine: Therapeutic touch. Nursing Times, 72, 572-4.

Kristiansen, C.M. (1984). Preventive Health Behaviour. Unpublished Doctoral Dissertation: University of Exeter.

Kronenfeld, J.J. and Wasner, C. (1982). The use of unorthodox therapies and marginal practitioners. Society of Scientific Medicine, 16, 1119-1125.

Kubler-Ross, E. (1969). On Death and Dying. New York: MacMillan.

Kuby, A. (1965). The Chiropractic Patient. Masters' Research Paper: University of Chicago.

Kupst, M.J., Presser, K., Schulman, J.L., and Paul, M.H. (1975). Evaluation of methods to improve communication in the physician-patient relationship. American Journal of Orthopsychology, 45, 420-429.

Langer, E.J. (1975). The illusion of control. Journal of Personality and Social Psychology, 32, 311-328.

Langer, E.J. (1977). The psychology of chance. Journal for the Theory of Social Behaviour, 7, 185-208.

Langer, E.J. (1983). The Psychology of Control. Sage.

Langlie, J.K. (1979). Interrelationships among preventive health behaviours: A test of competing hypotheses. Public Health Reports, 94, 216-225.

Lawson, N.C. (1976). Depression After Spinal Cord Injury: A Multi-Measure Longitudinal Study. Unpublished Doctoral Dissertation: University of Houston.

Lazarus, R.S. (1966). Psychological Stress and the Coping Process. New York: McGraw-Hill.

Lazarus, R.S. (1974). Psychological stress and coping in adaptation and illness.. Psychiatry in Medicine, 5, 321-333.

Lazarus, R.S. (1981). The stress and coping paradigm. In C. Eisdorfer, D. Cohen, A. Kleinman, and P. Maxim (Eds.), Models for Clinical Psychopathology. New York: Spectrum.

Lazarus, R.S. (1982). Stress and coping as factors in health and illness. In J. Cohen, J.W. Cullen, and L.R. Martin (Eds.), Psychosocial Aspects of Cancer. New York: Raven Press.

Lazarus, R.S., Averill, J.R., and Opton, E.M. Jr. (1974). The Psychology of coping: Issues of research and assessment. In G.V. Coelho, D.A. Hamburg, and J.E. Adams (Eds.), Coping and Adaptation. New York: Basic Books.

Lazarus, R.S. and Launier, R. (1978). Stress related transactions between person and environment. In L.A. Pervin and M. Lewis (Eds.), Perspectives in Interactional Psychology. New York: Plenum.

Leif, H.I. and Fox, R.C. (1963). Training for detached concern in medical students. In H.I. Lief (Ed.), The Psychological Basis of Medical Practice. New York: Harper and Row. Leslie, C. (1974). The modernization of Asian medical systems. In J. Poggie and R.N. Lynch (Eds.), Rethinking Modernization: Anthropological Perspectives. London: Greenwood Press.

Levenson, H. (1973). Multidimensional locus of control in psychiatric patients. Journal of Consulting and Clinical Psychology, 41, 397-404.

Leventhal, H., Brown, D., Shacham, S., and Engquist, G. (1979). Effects of preparatory information about sensations, threat of pain and attention on cold pressor distress. Journal of Personality and Social Psychology, 37, 688-714.

Levine, J. and Zigler, E. (1974). Denial and self-image in stroke, lung cancer and heart disease patients. Journal of Consulting and Clinical Psychology, 43, 751-757.

Levy, J.M. and McGee, R.K. (1975). Childbirth as crisis: A test of Janis' theory of commumication and stress resolution. Journal of Personality and Social Psychology, 31, 171-179.

Lewis-Faning, E. (1950). Report on an enquiry into the etiological factors associated with rheumatoid arthritis. Annals of the Rheumatic Diseases, 9 (Suppl.), 94.

Ley, P. (1972). Primacy, rated importance and the recall of medical information. Journal of Health and Social Behaviour, 13, 311-317.

Ley, P. (1974). Communication in the clinical setting. British Journal of Orthodontics 1, 173-177.

Ley, P. (1977). Psychological studies of doctor-patient communication. In S. Rachman (Ed.), Contributions to Medical Psychology, Volume I. Oxford: Pergamon Press.

Ley, P. (1979a). The psychology of compliance. In O.J. Oborne, M.M. Gruneberg, and J.R. Eiser (Eds.), Research in Psychology and Medicine, Volume II. Academic Press.

Ley, P. (1979b). Memory for medical information. British Journal of Social and Clinical Psychology, 18, 245-256.

Ley, P. (1982a). Giving information to patients. In J.R. Eiser (Ed.), Social Psychology and Behavioural Science. Wiley and Sons Limited.

Ley, P. (1982b). Studies of recall in medical settings. Human Learning, 1, 223-233.

Ley, P. (1983). Patients' understanding and recall in clinical communication failure. In P.D. Hasler, Doctor-Patient Communication. London: Academic Press.

Ley, P. (1985). Doctor-patient communication: Some quantitative estimates of the role of cognitive factors in non-compliance. Journal of Hypertension, 3 (Suppl.1), 51-55.

Ley, P., Bradshaw, P.W., Eaves, D., and Walker, C.M. (1973). A method for increasing patients' recall of information presented by doctors. Psychological Medicine, 3, 217-220.

Ley, P., Bradshaw, P.W., Kincey, J.A., and Atherton, S.T. (1976a). Increasing patients' satisfaction with communications. British Journal of Social and Clinical Psychology, 15, 403-413.

Ley, P., Bradshaw, P.W., Kincey, J.A., Comper-Smartt, J., and Wilson, M. (1974a). Psychological variables in the control of obesity. In W. Burland, P.D. Samuel, and J. Yudkin (Eds.), Obesity. London: Churchill Livingstone.

Ley, P., Goldman, M., Bradshaw, P.W., Kincey, J.A., and Walker, C. (1972). The comprehensibility of some x-ray leaflets. Journal of the Institute of Health Education, 10, 47-53.

Ley, P., Jain, V.K., and Skilbeck, C.E. (1975). A method for decreasing medication errors. Psychological Medicine, 6, 599-601.

Ley, P. and Morris, L.A. (1984). Psychological aspects of written information for patients. In S. Rachman (Ed.), Contributions to Medical Psychology: III. Oxford: Pergamon Press.

Ley, P. and Spelman, M.S. (1967). Communicating With The Patient. London: Staples Press.

Ley, P., Swinson, R., Bradshaw, P.W., and Kincey, J.A. (1974b). Satisfaction With Communication Amongst Surgical Patients. Unpublished manuscript - reported in Ley 1982.

Ley, P., Whitworth, M.A., Skilbeck, C.E., Woodward, R., Pinsent, R.J.F.H., Pike, L.A., Clarkson, M.E., and Clark, P.E. (1976b). Improving doctor-patient communications in general practice. Journal of the Royal College of General Practitioners, 26, 720-724.

Liang, M.H., Rogers, M., Larson, M., Eaton, H.M., Murawski, B.J., Taylor, J.E., Swafford, J., and Schur, P.H. (1984). The psychological impact of systemic lupus erythematosus and rheumatoid arthritis. Arthritis and Rheumatism, 27, 13-19.

Liguori, S. (1978). A quantitative assessment of the readability of PPIs. Drug Intelligence and Clinical Pharmacy, 12, 712-716.

Lipowski, Z.J. (1970). Physical illness, the individual and the coping process. Psychiatry in Medicine, 1, 91-102.

Logan, W.P.D. and Cushion A.A. (1958). Morbidity statistics from general practice. General Register Office, Studies on Medical and Population Subjects. No.14, vol.1.

Lorig, K. and Fries, J.E. (1980). Arthritis Help Book: What You Can Do For Your Arthritis. Addison-Wesley.

Lorig, K., Kraines, R.G., Byron, M.S., Brown, W.M. and Richardson, N. (1985a). A workplace health education program that reduces out-patient visits. Medical Care, 23, 1044-54.

Lorig, K., Laurin, J., and Holman, H.R. (1984). Arthritis self-management: A study of the effectiveness of patient education for the elderly. The Gerontologist, 24, 455-257.

Lorig, K., Lubeck, D., Kraines, R.G., Seleznick, M., and Holman, H.R. (1985b). Outcomes of self-help education for patients with arthritis. Arthritis and Rheumatism, 28, 680-685.

Lorish, C.D., Parker, J., and Brown, S. (1985). Effective patient education: A quasi-experiment comparing an individualized strategy with a routinized strategy. Arthritis and Rheumatism, 28, 1289-1297.

Lowery, B., Jacobsen, B., and Keane, A. (1975). Relationship of locus of control to pre-operative anxiety. Psychological Reports, 37, 1115-1121.

Ludwig, A.O. (1952). Psychogenic factors in rheumatic disease. Bulletin on the Rheumatic Diseases, 2, 15-16.

Ludwig, A.O. (1954). Rheumatoid arthritis. In E. Whittkower and R.A. Cleghorn, Recent Developments in Psychosomatic Medicine. Philadelphia: Lippincott.

Maddocks, J. (1985). Alternative medicine. The Medical Journal of Australia, 142, 547-551.

Maguire, G.P. and Rutter, D.R. (1976). History taking for medical students: 1. Deficiencies in performance. Lancet, 2, 556-558.

Maslow, A.H. (1954). Motivation and Personality. New York: Harper and Row.

Mason, R.M., Barnardo, D.E., Fox, W.R., and Weatherall, M. (1967). Assessment of drugs in out-patients with rheumatoid arthritis. Annals of the Rheumatic Diseases, 26, 373-388.

Mathews, A. and Ridgeway, V. (1984). Psychological preparation for surgery. In A. Steptoe and A. Mathews, Health Care and Human Behaviour. London: Academic Press.

Matson, R.R. and Brooks, N.A. (1979). Adjusting to multiple sclerosis: An exploratory study. Social Science and Medicine, 11, 245-250.

Mazzullo, J.M., Cohn, K., Lasagna, L., and Griner, P.F. (1974). Variations in interpretation of prescription instructions. Journal of the American Medical Association, 227, 929-931.

McAnarney, E., Pless, I.B., Satterwhite, B., and Friedman, S. (1974). Psychological problems of children with chronic juvenile arthritis. Pediatrics, 53, 523-528.

McCorkle, T. (1961). Chiropractic: A deviant theory of disease and treatment in contemporary Western culture. Human Organization, 20, 20-22.

McFie, J. and Robertson, J. (1973). Psychological test results of children with thalidomide disorders. Developmental Medicine and Child Neurology, 15, 719-727.

McKenny, J.M., Slining, J.M., Henderson, H.R., Devine, D, Barr, M., Stern, M.P., Farquar, J.W., Maccoby, N., and Russell, S.H. (1973). The effect of clinical pharmacy services on patients with essential hypertension. Circulation, 48, 1104-1111.

McLaughlin, J.T., Zabarenko, R.N., Diana, P.B., and Quinn, B. (1953). Emotional reactions of rheumatoid arthritics to ACTH. Psychosomatic Medicine, 15, 187-199.

Meenan, R.F., Gertman, P.M., and Mason, J.H. (1980). Measuring health status in arthritis: The Arthritis Impact Measurement Scales. Arthritis and Rheumatism, 23, 146-152.

Melzack, R. (1975). The McGill Pain Questionnaire: Major properties and scoring methods. Pain, 1, 277-299.

Melzack, R. and Wall, P.D. (1965). Pain mechanisms: A new theory. Science, 150, 971-979.

Meyerowitz, B.E. (1980). Psychological correlates of breast cancer and its treatments. Psychological Bulletin, 87, 108-131.

Meyerowitz, B.E. (1983). Post-mastectomy coping strategies and quality of life. Health Psychology, 2, 117-132.

Midgley, J.M. and Macrae, A.W. (1971). Audio-visual media in general practice. Journal of the Royal College of General Practitioners, 21, 346-351.

Miller, N.E. (1948). Studies of fear as an aquirable drive: 1. Fear as motivation and fear-reduction as reinforcement in the learning of new responses. Journal of Experimental Psychology, 38, 89-101.

Mindam, R.H.S., Bagshaw, A., James, S.A., and Swannel, A.J. (1981). Factors associated with the appearance of psychiatric symptoms in rheumatoid arthritis. Journal of Psychosomatic Research, 5, 429-435.

Mitchell, G.D. (1980). Introduction to Sociology: Magic, Religion and Society. Lecture presented to first year undergraduates. University of Exeter.

Moldofsky, H. and Rothman, A.I. (1971). Personality, disease parameters and medication in rheumatoid arthritis. Journal of Chronic Diseases, 24, 363-372.

Moos, R.H. and Engel, B.T. (1962). Psychophysiological reactions in hypertensive and arthritic patients. Journal of Psychosomatic Research, 6, 227-241.

Moos, R.H. and Solomon, G.F. (1964). Minnesota Multiphasic Personality Inventory response patterns in patients with rheumatoid arthritis. Journal of Psychosomatic Research, 8, 17.

Moos, R.H. and Solomon, G.F. (1965). Psychologic comparisons between women with rheumatoid arthritis and their non-arthritic sisters. Psychosomatic Medicine, 27, 135-164.

Morris, L.A. and Halperin, J. (1979). Effects of written drug information on patient knowledge and compliance: A literature review. American Journal of Public Health, 69, 47-52.

Mowrer, O.H. (1947). On the dual nature of learning - a reinterpretation of 'conditioning' and 'problem-solving'. Harvard Educational Review, 17, 102-148.

Mueller, A.D., Lefkovits, A.M., Bryant, J.E., and Marshall, M.L. (1961). Some psychosocial factors in patients with rheumatoid arthritis. Arthritis and Rheumatism, 4, 275-282.

Myers, E.D. and Calvert, E.J. (1973). Effects of the forewarning on the occurrence of side-effects and discontinuance of medication in patients on amitriptyline. British Journal of Psychiatry, 122, 461-464.

Myers, E.D. and Calvert, E.J. (1978). Knowledge of side-effects and perseverance with medication. British Journal of Psychiatry, 132, 526-527.

Natterson, J.M. and Knudson, A.G. (1960). Observations concerning fear of death in fatally ill children and their mothers. Psychosomatic Medicine, 22, 456-465.

Nichols, K.N. (1983). Medicine and the infallibility myth. The Guardian, 4th May.

Nichols, K.N. (1984). Psychological Care in Physical Illness. Beckenham, Kent: Croom Helm Limited.

Nighswonger, C.A. (1971). Ministry to the dying as a learning encounter. Journal of Thanatology, 1, 101-108.

Nugent, C.A., Ward, J., and MacDairmid, W.D. (1965). Glucocorticoid toxicity: Single contrasted with divided daily doses of prednisolone. Journal of Chronic Diseases, 18, 323-332.

Nunally, J.C. (1978). Psychometric Theory (2nd ed.). New york: McGraw-Hill.

Oppenheim, A.N. (1968). Questionnaire Design and Attitude Measurement. London: Heinemann.

Palmblad, J. (1981). Stress and immunologic competence: Studies in man. In R. Adler (Ed.), Psychoimmunology. New York: Academic Press.

Parker, G. (1975). Psychological disturbance in Darwin evacuees following Cyclone Tracey. Medical Journal of Australia, 1, 650-652.

Parker, G. and Tupling, H. (1976). The chiropractic patient - Psychosocial aspects. The Medical Journal of Australia, 2, 373-376.

Parker, J., Lorish, C., and Brown, S. (1984). An individualized rheumatoid arthritis education program: A case study. Arthritis and Rheumatism (Suppl.), 27, S132.

Parkes, C.M. (1972). Components of the reaction to loss of a limb, spouse or home. Journal of Thanatology, 1, 101-108.

Parkin, D.M. (1976). Survey of the success of communications between hospital staff and patients. Public Health (London), 90, 203-209.

Parsons, T. (1951). The Social System. New York: Free Press.

Paulson, P.T., Bauch, R., Paulson, M.L., and Zilz, D.A. (1976). Medication data sheets - an aid to patient education. Drug Intelligence and Clinical Pharmacy, 10, 448-453.

Pendleton, D.A. and Bochner, S. (1980). The communication of medical information in general practice consultations as a function of patients' social class. Social Science and Medicine, 14A, 669-673.

Pickering, P.M. (1986). Psychosocial Characteristics of Long-Term Tranquilliser Users, Unpublished Doctoral Dissertation: University of Exeter.

Plaja, A. and Cohen, S. (1968). Communication between physicians and patients in out-patient clinics: Social and cultural factors. Milbank Memorial Fund Quarterly, 46, 161-213.

Plaut, S.M. and Friedman, S.E. (1981). Psychosocial factors in infectious diseases. In R. Adler (Ed.) Psychoneuroimmunology. New York: Academic Press.

Podell, R.N. (1975). Physicians Guide to Compliance in Hypertension. New Jersey: Merck Rathway.

Polley, H.F., Swenson, W.M., and Steinhilber, R.M. (1970). Personality characteristics of patients with rheumatoid arthritis. Psychosomatics, 11, 45-49.

Prieto, E.J. and Geisinger, K.F. (1983). Factor - analytic studies of the McGill Pain Questionnaire. In R. Melzack, Pain Measurement and Assessment. New York: Raven Press.

Pruyn, J.F.A., Rijckman, R.M., Van Brunschot, C.J.M., and Van Den Borne, H.W. (1985). Cancer patients' personality characteristics, physician-patient communication and adoption of the Moerman diet. Social Science and Medicine, 20, 841-847.

Pyrezak, R. and Rotn, D.H. (1976). The readability of directions on non-prescription drugs. Journal of the American Pharmaceutical Association, 16, 242-243 and 267.

Ragan, C. (1949). General management of rheumatoid arthritis. Journal of the American Medical Association, 141, 124-127.

Ragan, C. and Farrington, E. (1962). The clinical features of rheumatoid arthritis. Prognostic indices. Journal of the American Medical Association, 181, 663.

Randich, S.R. (1982). Evaluation of a pain management program for rheumatoid arthritis patients (Abstract). Arthritis and Rheumatism, 25, S11.

Raphael, W. and Peers, V. (1972) Psychiatric Patients View Their Hospitals. King Edward's Hospital Fund, London.

Reading, A.E. (1983). The McGill Pain Questionnaire: An appraisal. In R. Melzack, Pain Measurement and Assessment. New York: Raven Press.

Reah, T.G. (1963). The prognosis of rheumatoid arthritis (183 patients followed-up over 13 years). Proceedings of the Royal Society of Medicine, 56, 813.

Rees, C.A. and Soheed, M.A. (1975). Agranulocytosis caused by Chinese herbal medicine. Journal of the American Medical Association, 231, 352-355.

Reichman, F. and Levy, N.B. (1972). Problems in adaptation to maintenance hemodialysis. Archives of Internal Medicine, 130, 859-865.

Relman, A.S. (1979). Chiropractic - recognized but unproved. New England Journal of Medicine, 301, 659.

Reynolds, P.M., Sanson-Fisher, R.W., Harker, J., and Byrne, M.J. (1979). Towards Improved Doctor-Patient Communications: Back To Basics. Mimeo, Sir Charles Gairdner Hospital, Western Australia.

Richards, J.S. (1980). Sex and arthritis. Sexuality and the Disabled, 3, 97-104.

Rigby, B. (1975). Alternative medicine: Transcendental meditation. Nursing Times, 71, 1240-1242.

Riley, C.S. (1966). Patients' understanding of doctors' instructions. Medical Care, 4, 34-37.

Riley, J.N. (1980). Client choices among osteopaths and ordinary physicians in a Michigan community. Social Science and Medicine, 14, 111-120.

Rimon, R. (1969). A psychosomatic approach to rheumatoid arthritis: A clinical study of 100 patients. Acta Rheumatologica Scandinavica Supplement, 13, 1-154.

Rimon, R. (1974). Depression in rheumatoid arthritis. Annals of Clinical Research, 6, 171-175.

Robinson, C.E. (1957). Emotional factors and rheumatoid arthritis. Canadian Medical Association Journal, 77, 344-345.

Robinson, H., Kirk, R.F., and Frye, R.L. (1971). A psychological study of rheumatoid arthritis and selected controls. Journal of Chronic Diseases, 23, 791-801.

Roessler, R. and Engel, B.T. (1974). The current status of the concept of physiological response specificity and activation. International Journal of Psychiatry in Medicine, 5, 359-366.

Rodda, M. (1970). The Hearing Impaired School Leaver. London: University of London Press.

Rogers, M.P., Liang, M.H., and Partridge, A.J. (1982). Psychological care of adults with rheumatoid arthritis. Annals of Internal Medicine, 96, 344-345.

Rose-Neil, S. (1976). Alternative medicine: Acupuncture. Nursing Times, 72, 687-689.

Rosenman, R.H., Braud, R.J., Jenkins, C.D., Friedman, M., Straus, R., and Wurm, M. (1975). Coronary heart disease in the Western Collaborative Group Study: Final follow-up experience of 8.5 years. Journal of the American Medical Association, 233, 872-877.

Rosenstock, I.M. (1966). Why people use health services. Milbank Memorial Fund Quarterly, 44, 94-127.

Roskam, S.E. (1986). Applications of a Health Locus of Control Typology Approach Towards Predicting Depression and Adherence in Rheumatoid Arthritis. Unpublished Doctoral Dissertation: Vanderbuilt University.

Roter, D.L. (1977). Patient participation in the patient-provider interaction: the effects of patient question-asking on the quality of interaction satisfaction and compliance. Health Education Monographs, 5, 281-315.

Rotter, J.B. (1954). Social Learning and Clinical Psychology. New York: Prentice Hall Inc.

Rotter, J.B. (1966). Generalized expectancies for internal versus external control of reinforcement. Psychological Monographs, 80, (Whole No.609).

Rotter, J.B. (1982). Social learning theory. In N.T. Feather (Ed.), Expectations and Actions: Expectancy- Value Models in Psychology. Hillsdale, New Jersey: Lawrence Erlbaum.

Rutter, M. and Quinton, D. (1976). Psychiatric disorder - Ecological factors and concepts of causation. In H. McGurk (Ed.), Ecological Factors in Human Development. Amsterdam: North Holland.

Rutter, M., Yule, B., Quinton, D., Rowlands, O., Yules, W., and Berger, M. (1975). Attainment and adjustment in two geographical areas: III. Some factors accounting for area differences. British Journal of Psychiatry, 126, 520-533.

Sackett, D.L., Haynes, R.B., Gibson, E.S., Hachet, B.C., Taylor, D.W., Roberts, R.S., and Johnson, A.L. (1975). Randomized clinical trials of strategies for improving medication compliance in primary hypertension. Lancet, 1, 1205-1207.

Salmon, J.W. (Ed.) (1984). Alternative Medicines: Popular and Policy Perspectives. London: Tavistock Publications.

Saltzer, E.B. (1979). Casual Beliefs and Losing Weight: A Study of Behavioural Intention Theory and Locus of Control in Prediction of Health-Related Behaviour. Unpublished Doctoral Dissertation: University of California at Irvine.

Schafer, L.C., Russell, M.S., Glasgow, E., McCaul, K.D., and Dreher, M. (1983). Adherence to IDDM regimens: Relationship to psychosocial variables and metabolic control. Diabetes Care, 6, 493-498.

Schmitt, M.H. (1978). The utilization of chiropractors. Sociological Symposium, 22, 55-74.

Schwartz, L.R. (1969). The hierarchy of resort in curative practices. Journal of Health and Social Behaviour, 10, 201-298.

Schwartz, L.H., Marcus, R., and Condon, R. (1978). Multidisciplinary group therapy for rheumatoid arthritis. Psychosomatics, 19, 289-293.

Scott, J. and Huskisson, E.C. (1979). Vertical on horizontal visual analogue scales. Annals of the Rheumatic Diseases, 38, 560.

Seligman, M.E.P. (1975). Helplessness: On Depression, Development and Death. San Francisco: W.H. Freeman.

Seligman, M.E.P. and Maier, S.F. (1967). Failure to escape traumatic shock. Journal of Experimental Psychology, 74, 1-9.

Shepherd, M., Cooper, B., Brown, A.C., and Kalton, G.W. (1966). Psychiatric Illness in General Practice. London: Oxford University Press.

Shontz, F.C. (1965). Reactions to crisis. The Volta Review, 67, 364-370.

Shontz, F.C. (1975). The Psychological Aspects of Physical Illness and Disability. New York: Macmillan.

Shuy, R. (1974). Problems of communication in the cross-cultural medical interview. Working papers: Sociolinguistics 19, Washington, DC. Mimeo.

Siller, J. (1969). Psychological situation of the disabled with spinal cord injuries. Rehabilitation Literature, 30, 290-296.

Silver, R.L. and Wortman, C.B. (1980). Coping with undesirable life events. In J. Garber and M.E.P. Seligman, Human Helplessness. London: Academic Press.

Sime, A.M. (1976). Relationship of pre-operative fear, type of coping and information received about surgery to recovery from surgery. Journal of Personality and Social Psychology, 34, 716-724.

Skevington, S.M. (in press). A standardised scale to measure beliefs about controlling pain. Psychology and Health.

Smith, R.T. and Midanik, L. (1980). The effect of social resources on recovery and perceived sense of control among the disabled. Sociology of Health and Illness, 2, 48-63.

Snellgrove, B. (1976). Alternative medicine: Kirlian photography. Nursing Times, 72, 571.

Sochet, B.R., Lisansky, E.T., Schubart, A.F., Fiocco, V., Kurland, S., and Pope, M. (1969). A medical-psychiatric study of patients with rheumatoid arthritis. Psychosomatics, 10, 271-279.

Solomon, G.F. (1981). Emotional and personality factors in the onset and course of autoimmune disease, particularly rheumatoid arthritis. In R. Adler (Ed.), Psychoneuroimmunology. New York: Academic Press.

Spector, H.N. and Korneva, E.A. (1981). Neurophysiological, immunophysiology and neuroimmunomodulation. In R. Adler (Ed.), Psychoimmunology. New York: Academic Press.

Spergel, P., Ehrlich, G.E., and Glass, D. (1978). The rheumatoid arthritic personality: A psychodiagnostic myth. Psychosomatics, 19, 79-86.

Steinbrocker, O., Traeger, C.H., and Batterman, R.C. (1949). Therapeutic criteria in rheumatoid arthritis. Journal of the American Medical Association, 140, 659.

Sternbach, R.A. (1966). Principles of Psychophysiology. New York: Academic Press.

Stourkes, B. (1982). The Deepening Shade: Psychological Aspects of Life-Threatening Illness. Pittsburgh: Union of Pittsburgh Press.

Sussman, M.B. (1966). Sociological theory and deafness: Problems and prospects. ASHA: Journal of the American Speech and Hearing Association, 8, 303-307.

Sutherland, S. and Scherl, D. (1970). Patterns of response among victims of rape. American Journal of Orthopsychiatry, 40, 503-511.

Suveges, L. (1977). The Impact of Counselling by the Pharmacist on Patient Knowledge and Compliance. Procedings of the McMaster symposium on compliance with therapeutic regimens. Mcmaster University, Hamilton, Ontario.

Svarstad, B.L. (1974). The Doctor-Patient Encounter. Unpublished Doctoral Dissertation: University of Wisconsin.

Svarstad, B.L. (1976). Physician-patient communication and patient conformity with medical advice. In D. Mechanic (Ed.), The Growth of Bureaucratic Medicine: An Inquiry into the Dynamics of Patient Behaviour and the Organization of Medical Care. New York: Wiley.

Syme, S.L. and Berkman, L.F. (1976). Social class, susceptibility and sickness. American Journal of Epidemiology, 104, 1-8.

Symonds, M. (1975). Victims of violence: Psychological effects and after effects. The American Journal of Psychoanalysis, 35, 19-26.

Szasz, T. and Hollander, M. (1956). A contribution to the philosophy of medicine: The basic models of the doctor-patient relationship. Archives of Internal Medicine, 97, 585-592.

Taylor, D.W. (1979). A test of the health belief model in hypertension. In R.B. Haynes, D.W. Taylor, and D.L. Sackett (Eds.), Compliance in Health Care. Baltimore: John Hopkins University Press.

Taylor, J.A., Gatchel, R.J., and Korman, M. (1982). Psychophysiological and cognitive characteristics of ulcer and rheumatoid arthritis patients. Journal of Behavioural Medicine, 5, 173-188.

Taylor, W.M. (1978). Schizophrenia, rheumatoid arthritis and trytophan metabolism. Journal of Clinical Psychiatry, 39, 499-502.

Thoits, P.A. (1982). Conceptual, methodological and theoretical problems in studying social support as a buffer against life stress. Journal of Health and Social Behaviour, 23, 145-159.

Thompson, S.C. (1981). Will it hurt less if I can control it? A complex answer to a simple question. Psychological Bulletin, 90, 89-101.

Thurstone, L.L. (1947). Multiple Factor Analysis. University of Chicago Press.

Tolman, E.C. (1955). Principles of performance. Psychological Review, 62, 315-326.

Townsend, P. and Davidson, N. (1982). Inequalities in Health. Harmondsworth: Penguin Books Limited.

Tversky, A. and Kahneman, D. (1977). Judgements under uncertainty: Heuristics and bias. Science, 185, 1124, 1131.

Udelman, H.D. and Udelman, D.L. (1981). Emotions and rheumatological disorders. American Journal of Psychotherapy, 35, 576-587.

Udelman, H.D. and Udelman, D.L. (1983). Current exploration in psychoimmunology. American Journal of Psychotherapy, 37, 210-221.

Vignos, P., Parker, W.T., and Thompson, H.M. (1976). Evaluation of a clinical education program for patients with rheumatoid arthritis. Journal of Rheumatology, 3, 155-165.

Vissing, Y.M. and Peterson, J.C. (1981). Talking laetrile: Conversion to medical deviance. Ca: A Cancer Journal for Clinicians, 31, 365-369.

Waitzkin, H. and Stoeckle, J.D. (1972). The communication of the information about illness. Advances in Psychosomatic Medicine, 8, 180.

Walker, B.B. and Sandman, C.A. (1977). Physiological response patterns in ulcer patients: Phasic and tonic components of the electrogastrogram. Psychophysiology, 14, 393-400.

Wallston, B.S., Wallston, K.A., Kaplan, G.D., and Maides, S.A. (1976). Development and validation of the health locus of control (HLC) scale. Journal of Consulting and Clinical Psychology, 44, 580-585.

Wallston, K.A. and Wallston, B.S. (1982). Who is responsible for your health? The construct of health locus of control. In G. Sanders and J. Suls (Eds.), Social Psychology of Health and Illness. Hillside, New Jersey: Erlbaum.

Wallston, K.A., Wallston, B.S., and DeVellis, R. (1978). Development of the Multidimensional Health Locus of Control Scales. Health Education Monographs, 6, 160-171.

Walrad, R. (1960). The Misrepresentation of Arthritis Drugs and Devices in the United States. Arthritis and Rheumatism Foundation.

Wardwell, W.I. (1951). Social Strain and Social Adjustment in the Marginal Role of the Chiropractor. Unpublished Doctoral Dissertation: Harvard University.

Wasner, C., Britton, M.C., and Kraines, R.G. (1981). Non-steroidal anti-inflammatory agents in rheumatoid arthritis and ankylosing spondilitus. Journal of the American Medical Association, 246, 2168-2172.

Webb, B. (1976). The retail pharmacist and drug treatment. Journal of the Royal College of General Practitioners, 26, Supplement 1, 81-88.

Weibert, R.T. (1977). Potential distribution problems. Drug Information Journal, 11, (Special Supplement), 45-48.

Weiner, H. (1977). Psychobiology and Human Disease. New York: Elsevier.

Weiss, R.S. (1974). The provisions of social relationships. In Z. Rubin (Ed.), Doing Unto Others. Engle Wood Cliffs, New Jersey: Prentice Hall.

Weissman, M.M. and Myers, J.K. (1978). Rates and risks of depressive disorders in a US suburban community. Acta Psychiatrica Scandinavica, 57, 219-231.

Weller, D.J. and Miller, P.M. (1977). Emotional reactions of patient, family and staff in acute-care period of spinal cord injury: Part 1. Social Work in Health Care, 2, 369-377.

Westbrook, M.T. and Viney, L.L. (1982). Psychological reactions to the onset of chronic illness. Social Science and Medicine, 16, 899-905.

Wetstone, S.L., Sheehan, Votaw, R., and Peterson, M. (1982). Computer-based education in rheumatoid arthritis. Arthritis and Rheumatism (Suppl.), 25, 526.

White, R.L. and Liddon, S.C. (1972). Ten survivors of cardiac arrest. Psychiatry in Medicine, 3, 219-225.

Wilcox, J. (1976). Alternative medicine: Radionics. Nursing Times, 72, 568-570.

Williams, C. (1970). Some psychiatric observations on a group of maladjusted deaf children. Journal of Child Psychiatry and Allied Disciplines, 11, 1-18.

Wing, J.K. (1976). A technique for studying psychiatric morbidity in in-patient and out-patient series and in general population samples. Psychological Medicine, 6, 665-672.

Wolinsky, F.D. (1980). The Sociology of Health. Boston, MA: Little, Brown and Co.

Wortman, C.B. and Brehm, J.W. (1975). Responses to uncontrollable outcomes: An integration of reactance theory and the learned helplessness model. In L. Berkowitz (Ed.), Advances in Experimental Social Psychology, (Vol.8). New York: Academic Press.

Yelin, E., Feshbach, D.M., Meenan, R.F., and Epstein, W.V. (1979). Social problems, services and policy for persons with chronic disease: The case of rheumatoid arthritis. Social Science and Medicine, 13, 13-20.

Yesalis, C.E., Wallace, R.B., Fisher, W.P., and Tokheim, R. (1980). Does chiropractic utilization substitute for less available medical services? American Journal of Public Health, 70, 4-15.

Zahourek, R. and Jensen, J.S. (1973). Grieving and the loss of the newborn. American Journal of Nursing, 73, 836-839.

Zaphiropoulos, G. and Burry, H.C. (1974). Depression in rheumatoid disease. Annals of the Rheumatic Diseases, 33, 132-135.

Zimmerman, M. (1983). Methodological issues in the assessment of life events: A review of issues and research. Clinical Psychology Review, 3, 339-370.

Zung, W. (1965). A self-rating depression scale. Archives of General Psychiatry, 12, 63-70.